FULL HEART LIVING

FULL
HEART
LIVING

Conversations with the Happiest People I Know

Tom Glaser

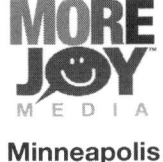

Minneapolis

MoreJoy Media
www.fullheartliving.com
1409 Willow Street
Suite 400
Minneapolis, MN 55403

ISBN: 978-0-9861333-3-6

Cover design: Kathi Dunn, dunn-design.com
Interior design: Dorie McClelland, springbookdesign.com

Second printing.

Dedication

To Greg and Elliot, who continue to surprise and delight me.
Thank you for your love and patience.

And to my parents. You made it all possible.

Contents

Epilogue: Thirteen Boulders in the Woods

NOTE TO READERS

Great loss, considerable confusion, and profound unhappiness—daily components of one of the most difficult periods in my adult life— propelled me to do the laborious work of deep soul searching. Who am I really? What is truly important to me? What do I most want to do in this life? In time, my efforts paid off and yielded unexpected gains and insight. I was inspired to seek out the happiest people I know, glean and collate their secrets, and then share what I learned. With ample use of quotes from these exceptionally happy people and examples from my own experiences, this book examines the everyday actions people make (and avoid making) to foster their happiness. It presents, in clear language, the themes I heard, including Taking Care of Yourself, Expressing Gratitude, Living Your Passion, Being Mindful, Developing Resilience, Giving Back, and more.

Some of the book's content may surprise you. It includes a number of less-than-pleasant stories, and your habits may be questioned. You might find yourself feeling challenged or uncomfortable at times. If such reactions occur, notice your thoughts and sensations. Take a deep breath, perhaps pause, and be with the fullness of your immediate experience. You may find that when you tune in and honor in this way, the arising judgments spontaneously lessen or even pass.

Readers of this book's earlier versions requested specific suggestions on how to bring the concepts into their own lives. Thus, each chapter ends with a section titled, "Putting It into Practice." I offer these exercises and action steps as ways for readers to go further and deepen their experience. Don't feel you have to complete all—or any—of them; just do those that most appeal to you. If you'd rather not write in the book, the activities and worksheets are available at www.fullheartliving.com.

As a psychologist and life coach, I use the term "client" to refer to an individual coming to me for psychotherapy or coaching. Client representations are composites of more than one person. I include them to illustrate concepts, and I have altered names, details, and distinguishing characteristics to prevent identification of particular individuals and to maintain confidentiality and protect privacy. Personal anecdotes are told to the best of my recollection, and some names and details therein have been changed or omitted to provide anonymity.

The term "interviewee" indicates a volunteer who agreed to a filmed interview regarding happiness. None of my interviewees are or were ever my psychotherapy or coaching clients. While all interviewee quotes are in the speaker's own words, some slight alterations not affecting the speaker's meaning were made for proper grammar and/or clarity.

Happier people are more apt to do good deeds. I sincerely hope that reading this book inspires you not just to be happier, but also to reach your highest potential and give back to your communities. If we all aim for that, I can't help but believe the world will be a happier, healthier place.

"When we feed and support our own happiness,
we are nourishing our ability to love.
That's why to love means to learn the art of nourishing our happiness."
~Thích Nhat Hanh, Beloved Vietnamese Buddhist Monk, *How to Love*

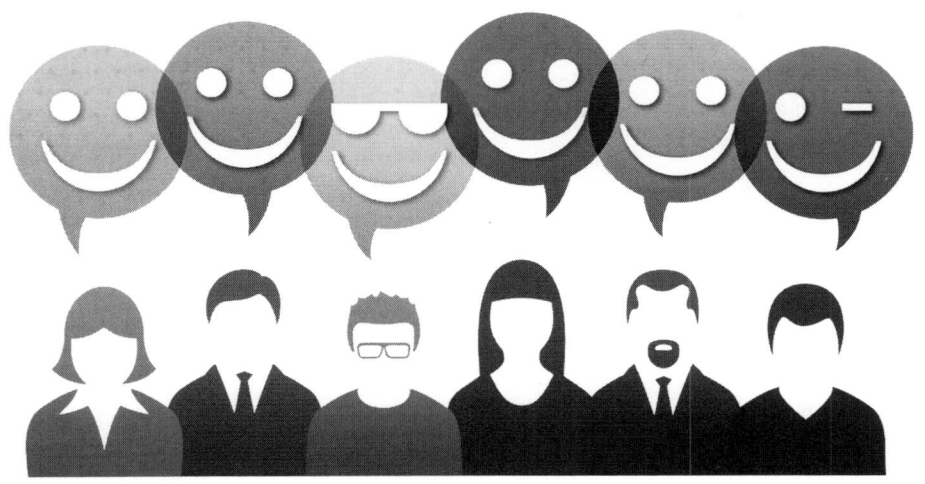

PART ONE

Before Happy

CHAPTER 1

Happiness lost:
Happiness found

Unhappiness can enter our lives in many ways. Sometimes the cause is obvious and dramatic, striking in one horrible moment when we learn that our life has been forever changed by an accident, death, illness, lay-off, divorce. Unhappiness can also seep in without notice. The only clue is a vague sensation that "something is off," that we are not living our best life. "Did I miss a turn somewhere? Get off at the wrong exit?" you might find yourself asking.

Still another kind of unhappiness falls somewhere in between. This kind of unhappiness takes a while to announce itself, mostly because we are desperately trying to ward it off. In my case, it began the day my boss introduced me to my new colleague. As the psychologist at a small college, a job I loved enormously, I spent half my time meeting individually with smart, talented, creative young people, helping them solve their problems. The other half of my time involved collaborating with a colleague to create wellness promotion activities to help students live healthier lives. For the prior seven years, I enjoyed a fantastic relationship with my former coworker. She and I developed a campus-wide reputation for producing effective, memorable, fun events.

The first two weeks with my new colleague went well. He smiled, made eye contact, listened, and contributed. I was sure there would be no problems between us. This made the abrupt change I was about to face all the more baffling. By the third week, my new colleague started ignoring me. When we passed in the hallway, he stared straight ahead as though he didn't see me. While it struck me as odd, I decided to ignore the behavior. Maybe he's just highly focused, I told myself, brushing off the unsettled feeling. Trying to foster a connection, I stopped by his office and made attempts at casual conversation. "How was your weekend?" I asked the next Monday. He stared at his computer screen. "It was good," he said in a monotone. He did not elaborate. He didn't ask me about my weekend. He continued typing as though I wasn't there.

By the fifth week, he began to miss important planning meetings. When I mentioned this, he acknowledged it with only a slight nod of his head and walked away. He then began to fail to reply to time-sensitive emails. And later, though he was in charge of the budget, he didn't pay key vendors on time. They contacted me, as I was the person they were familiar with. When I forwarded their complaints to him, my colleague emailed back a terse, one sentence reply: "I didn't have their addresses." This was puzzling, as I had provided their addresses to him weeks before, when we first agreed to host the event. (I had the email to prove it.) Nor did it explain why he didn't ask for the addresses if he couldn't find them. Hoping these were oversights of someone new to his job and not the beginning of a pattern, I chose not to mention these facts. Trying to be generous, I gave him the benefit of the doubt.

Happy people are big on giving others the benefit of the doubt. The problem is that our social generosity can make us easy marks. Worse, at weak moments, we start to doubt ourselves—am I doing something wrong? Why doesn't he like me? His relentless unpleasantness left me feeling shocked, puzzled, and uncertain. His predecessor and I had enjoyed a magnificent relationship. Working well with colleagues, in fact, was often noted on my performance reviews. What was wrong with me? Had I changed? Was I eating too much garlic? Finally, I tried talking with my new colleague directly. "Is there something we need to talk about?" I asked. "Anything I'm doing that's bothering you?" His head cocked to the side, his nose crinkled, and a puzzled expression covered his face. "No!" he replied, his tone implying I was crazy for asking. His utter dismissiveness left me so stunned that I failed to ask follow-up questions and quickly made up an excuse to leave. My confusion grew and eventually led to self-doubt. How much of this was him, and how much me?

Finally, I shared my list of concerns with our supervisor, who listened and sympathized but had little to suggest. More endlessly long weeks passed. Nothing changed. I returned to our supervisor. She sighed and said, "You're going to have to work this out on your own."

I got the message. I stopped asking my boss for help. Months went by. Things only got worse. I was left out of important meetings and events. When I was invited and it was my time to make a report, there was suddenly no room left on the agenda. Projects that were my colleague's ideas—or that involved no one else—went without a hitch. When others or I were on the team, however, he always complained that something was wrong. And somehow these errors never had anything to do with him.

I realize now that when dealing with a prickly, passive-aggressive coworker whose memory seems to favor only his side of the story, it is not uncommon to either blame yourself or think you are crazy. Thus, to counteract that, it is wise to always have another colleague present during any official meetings or interactions. A witness to his bad behavior would have helped me to see that it wasn't my fault and I wasn't insane.

I couldn't believe that after seven years of living my dream job and planning on working there until I retired, someone who had been there only half a year made me dread going to work. What was going on with me? How was it that one "toxic" co-worker could shake me up so badly?

I thought a lot about my history, trying to see if my reaction had its roots in my past. I found my eighth-grade English autobiography that I keep tucked away in a basement closet in a special bin full of childhood mementos. Its opening line reads, "I'm basically a happy person." Thirteen years old and I knew at my core that I'm happy! I had friends and a stable family, school was easy, and teachers liked me. But what astounds me now is that I wrote that after spending much of the previous year being tormented by bullies.

The bullying started when I made the mistake of wearing a green T-shirt with "Nags Head" printed in large white, block letters emblazoned across the chest. Nags Head is a beach community in North Carolina's Outer Banks, where my family and I had been for summer vacation. "Fag's head," said Merril, the first of many tormentors. "Fag's head, fag's head, fag's head," he hurled the words, his volume increasing with every utterance. Soon a crowd formed. Pointing at me, a wicked smirk spread across Merril's twisted features. I wanted to disappear.

The word "Fag" was scrawled across my locker more times than I can remember. I was also called "Queer," "Wuss," "Pansy," "Ladies' man," and many more. On the bus, in the hallway, on the street—a confrontation could happen anywhere, anytime. "Watch out. We're gonna beat your gay ass," they jeered. I never was beaten up, but the threat of physical harm or verbal harassment was ever-present. I never knew when or where it might happen. Paranoia and anxiety were my constant companions. Thinking back, I wonder if this experience might have some relevance to the anxiety I'm feeling around my so-less-than-pleasant coworker.

Back in school, it didn't occur to me to tell the bullies off or ask an adult for help. Not only was I a fairly nonassertive kid, I had been taught both at home and in church that the best way to deal with such behavior is to ignore it. Responding in any way encourages and reinforces it, the theory goes. There's a lot to be said for that approach; many wise prophets advise it. While I do believe there is a time and place for turning the other cheek, what I've realized since, however, is that there is also a time to stand up for oneself, to demand to be treated with respect. Furthermore, only from a place of strength and confidence can one ignore abuse without harming oneself. At that point, young and sensitive, I was anything but strong. I was humiliated and deeply ashamed.

A common response to humiliation and shame (key fallouts from any trauma) is paralysis; it's the old fight, flight, or freeze response. I couldn't fight. I had nowhere to run. The only option I could summon was to freeze, overlook it as best I could, and hope with all my might that it would stop. But such hopes were in vain. The bullying continued unabated for the next three years.

What saved me was theater. I was wild about performing. I loved the focus, the creativity, the teamwork, the artistic expression, the challenge of inhabiting another person's mannerisms and expressions. To me, it was all magic. There, in a world of creative, open, funny souls—many of them misfits like myself—I blossomed. I felt at home. I had fun. I was well liked for being who I was. From that first production of *The King and I*, I was almost constantly on stage. Having something I excelled at and a setting in which I made friends saved me.

I thought long and hard about bullies and the profound effect they can have on others. I was living proof that trauma has a long shelf life. But then I realized what saved me in junior high and high school just might help me now. I needed to get back to what truly made me happy: performing. I didn't know how I would do that, but it was a start. Just thinking about it lifted my mood. Meanwhile, I still had to deal with my horrendous work situation.

Deep down, I suspected there was no fixing this job. And so on one cold, grey Minnesota Sunday, my husband Greg and I were seated in the basement restaurant Hell's Kitchen in downtown Minneapolis. It was a rare moment for us to dine out without our young son in tow. While waiting for our food, I told Greg about the latest escapade at work. Once again, my nemesis coworker had misinterpreted something I'd said, and instead of coming to me, he went to our boss.

Greg interrupted my verbal ruminations. "Tom. This isn't working. You're miserable." (It occurred to me only later that, out of the kindness of his heart, Greg left out the part about how miserable I was making *him*.) "If you want to leave, just leave. This is not worth it."

I listened. When Greg had suggested this before, I wouldn't hear of it. I wasn't going to quit my dream job—at least not lightly. But then it began to dawn on me. My colleague was not going to change. I thought I could wait him out and that he'd soon get a job elsewhere. But he was not going anywhere. About half my job (the part he's not involved in), where I worked individually doing psychotherapy with students, I still felt tremendous passion for. The other half, which used to bring me great joy, I now dreaded. With half my job enjoyable and half bringing frustration and misery, the two canceled each other out. I could live with an 80:20, or perhaps even a 70:30, but a 50:50 ratio just doesn't cut it.

It's like a light bulb popped on. I need to prepare! With my husband's full support, I knew I could be happy in my work again. An idea started forming—why not go into private practice? With Greg's words fresh in my mind, I went from surviving day to day to planning my escape.

A big reason I became a psychologist in the first place was that I was so intrigued and jazzed to study the work of Abraham Maslow, one of the first psychologists to make the radical claim that we could benefit not only from examining mental dysfunctions, but also from studying those people who are functioning well. With his theory of self-actualization, Maslow emphasized the importance of focusing on the positive qualities in people, as opposed to treating them as a "bag of symptoms." When the Positive Psychology movement, spearheaded by Martin Seligman, made headlines years later, I was an early adopter. I naturally found myself actively doing all sorts of things to be happy. I got into exercise. I ate a mostly vegetarian diet. I studied with a Native American spiritual teacher, the Venerable Dhyani Ywahoo. I learned to meditate. To work through the craziness in my family and heal from the trauma of being bullied, I found myself a good therapist. I began to define myself as a survivor instead of as a victim. Why not see if I could help others focus on finding the positive in their lives?

When we make a shift to embrace our true selves, the universe often bestows gifts. Just before quitting my job, I stumbled upon a book that rocked my world. In *The Happiness Project*, author Gretchen Rubin writes about loving her work as a freelance journalist in New York City. She had a devoted husband and two adorable girls. Like many

Americans, Rubin was living the good life. But something was missing. She knew she could be happier. *The Happiness Project* tells the tale of the inspiring year she spent researching happiness, and the simple, straightforward steps she took applying what she learned.

Reading *The Happiness Project* propelled and galvanized me. It struck me that happiness entails areas I studied—and loved—for years: mindfulness, positive psychology, wellness, emotional intelligence, and resilience. In addition to performing, I realized that what would make me happy is to share all I was learning and experiencing with others. Soon I found myself teaching classes on happiness, and I began wondering if there might be a way to fuse my two interests—the study and promotion of happiness and the performing arts.

After I quit my dream job, one thing I decided to do to make me happy was to get involved more in the arts—everything from performing to singing to video projects. And then it hit me; why not create a conversation about happiness? Nearly everyone says they want to be happy. But how many people can easily define what that even means to them? We seem to take it for granted, as though we'll just know when we get there. And who can't point to people who seem especially happy—but what specifically do we see in them? How do we know they're happy? And do they see the same things in themselves? What do happier people do that's different from the rest of us? Well, I became determined to find out.

I was studying with an on-camera acting coach, and one day, while leaving his studio, it occurred to me. I could produce a documentary on happiness—I could videotape interviews of happy people talking about being happy. I wanted to know how people obtain happiness and how they are able to maintain it. Had they always been happy? Did something happen in their life to wake them up to the need to be happy? How do they sustain happiness in tough times? I had a slew of questions.

I talked about my video project with my spouse, Greg. He loved the concept, but—always the voice of reason—he asked me, "How are you going to tell who's really happy?" He was right, of course. Did I have any criteria for what being happy is?

Good questions. I thought a lot about it. So did I know any truly happy people? What convinced me they're happy? While I wasn't necessarily aware of it on a conscious level at the time, I realize in retrospect I was drawn to those who had a sense of "positivity" about them. I found, too, in talking to potential candidates, that the people who seemed happier were hopeful and encouraging rather than complaining a lot or dwelling on the negative. They're also cheerful. Their faces are bright. Verbally and nonverbally, they engage with people. They're considerate, generous, and enthusiastic. They're loving and have big hearts. They show interest in other people and are engaged in activities they're passionate about. I was about to learn that being passionate about work and activities is a big key to happiness. When you enjoy what you do, it's far easier to make it through the parts of life that are more challenging.

One of the first things I asked my subjects is whether they see themselves as happy, and naturally, the ones I ended up choosing said yes. And for good measure (and to please my husband), I asked them to complete a few brief happiness inventories (see appendix). But I wasn't a stickler about them. There were no strict cut-off scores.

But as helpful as the happiness assessments were, they still felt somehow unsatisfying and incomplete. After some thought, I realized that my number one common denominator for happiness is that all the people I chose to interview make me laugh. I started to notice that I feel my spirits rise when I'm with them.

Here's an introduction to each of them. Nine of the happiest people I know:

Gretchen: "Real happiness is to be in a state of consciousness."

I met Gretchen, a recent college graduate, at an intense, three-week opera/music theater training program a few years ago. Because she's tall and slender with striking features and luxuriant, long brown hair, I noticed Gretchen right away. Her posture is superb, and she moves with a dancer's agile, breathtaking fluidity.

I learned later—no surprise—that she's a yoga instructor. But beyond her beauty and grace, it's Gretchen's gorgeous smile and contagious, ebullient laughter that most capture my attention. I feel good when I'm near her.

Plus, she's fully *her*. How do I explain it? Gretchen takes risks. She speaks her truth, even if some might think she's a bit "out there" (otherwise known as "quirky"). Gretchen loves to talk—and she has much to say, especially for someone in her mid-twenties. She travels the world to study with native spiritual teachers, and she likes to share her experiences. She teaches meditation, something I didn't feel comfortable doing until my 40s. Plus, she's so positive. In the music training program before rehearsal one day, Gretchen announced, "I love everything about this program! The teachers, the students, the material!" This is just one small example of her overflowing optimism. I started to wonder: Is she always smiling? I became determined to find out. Gretchen was happy to share her story on camera.

Warren: "I utilize a sense of awareness that I believe other people just do not take advantage of."

My friends Janet and Joel had long been telling me about their hairstylist of 20 years, Warren. They so love him that they drive 90 miles round-trip to get their haircuts each month.

I had passed by Warren's hair salon near uptown Minneapolis countless times. Conjuring up images of bloodshed and trickery, its name, "Sweeney Todd's," concerned me. But I needn't have worried. Warren is as light and funny as his salon's namesake is dark and serious. He has a very contented presence, and he loves to joke while he cuts hair.

"Everyone's entitled to my opinion," he might quip, followed quickly by, "If I wanted your opinion, I'd give it to you." His laughter resounds throughout the salon. I was impressed by his genuinely happy presence, especially since I had been told that Warren had gone through some very tough times before he opened his shop. I wanted to know how he got here from there. Without hesitating, he agreed to be my second subject.

Mia: "I feel really blessed that I have so much love in my life."

I first heard of Mia through her flyer, which I noticed tacked to the bulletin board at a local meditation center. Simple and elegant, in white font on black background, it read,

find balance.
make mindful choices.
enhance your life.
heal your pain.
be empowered.

Below that appeared, "Buddhist-inspired psychotherapy" along with Mia's name and business phone number.

I was impressed—and envious. I'd worked for months, wracking my brain to craft a statement that summed up my psychology practice. Mine was nowhere near as good. Mia created just the kind of ad I was after.

Turns out she had just moved to the vacant office right next to mine. I decided to leave her a note complimenting her on her flyer and inviting her to meet for coffee. I'll never forget seeing her breeze into Caribou, a coffee shop down the street. Her blond hair and the pastel colors she wore (and, I later learned, often wears) grabbed my attention right away. Instead of "Good Morning," she greeted the barista with a heartfelt, "Bon Jour!" We hit it off immediately. With her sweet smile and big heart, I found Mia open, friendly, safe, and inviting.

As only two introverts can, Mia and I dispensed with superficialities right off the bat. Meditation, feelings, group dynamics, and spiritual teachings are just a few of the topics we explored. Mia came to call me "Super Tom," which naturally led to my pet name for her, "Magnificent Mia." I feel loved in her presence. I learned more about how and why during her interview.

Philip: "Happiness is an anchoring force in my life. I'm almost ridiculously obsessive about the notion of being happy."

I adore the story of how I met Philip. One mild Thanksgiving weekend, I traveled to my childhood home. Needing exercise, my brother Joe and I headed out for a walk in downtown Rochester, Michigan. Passing South Street Skate Shop on Main Street, a T-shirt instantly caught my eye. "Detroit LIVES!" it boldly proclaimed. This sentiment is near and dear to my heart, as Detroit is the city of my birth, and it gets so much negative press. I'll be the first to admit that some of it is deserved, but much of it isn't. T-shirt in hand, I asked the storeowner about the artist. "He's young and local," she told me. "He lives in downtown Detroit," about 45 minutes to the south and east. "He's supposed to deliver more color choices sometime this weekend."

As if on cue, synchronicity strikes, and—I kid you not—in he walked. Smart and charming, with curly hair, perfect teeth, a few days' beard, and wearing jeans and a hoodie, Philip is much like the young artists with whom I so often work in coaching and psychotherapy. Our conversation was as comfortable as the jeans and sweatshirt he was wearing. Philip brimmed with enthusiasm for his art. I bought four shirts before bidding Philip a fond farewell. When I started my video project, I thought of Philip and the strong impression he made, and I was able to track him down on the Internet without too much effort. I was afraid he wouldn't remember me or wouldn't be interested in my happiness quest. I was wrong on both counts. "I'll do it," he offered generously. With my parents and two siblings living nearby, Philip and I made plans to meet at his workplace in Detroit the next time I was to be in Michigan. I hoped to find out how Philip came to be so upbeat.

Barry: "I'm hopelessly optimistic. And naturally caffeinated."

I met Barry in Indianapolis at a national conference for counseling center directors. Though it's a casual gathering, most attendees dressed up a bit, wearing pants and long-sleeved shirts. It was November, after all. Barry wore shorts. I came to learn this is the epitome of Barry. Not worrying about what others do or think, he does what's right for him. He's tall, muscular, and what remains of his hair is thick and unruly. His soft blue eyes provide steady, reassuring, unwavering eye contact. I felt an instant connection. I was truly happy to see him at subsequent conferences. I was impressed by how much he values happiness in every walk of his life. Fortunately Barry lived near my sister in Connecticut. When I was out visiting her, I made plans to swing by Barry's inviting New England home. Subject five, booked.

Ryan: "Happiness is doing what you love."

Ryan, a local filmmaker, is one of the organizers of Minneapolis' 48 Hour Film Project. In this insomnia-inducing event, teams have just two days to complete an entire short film. I'm not sure if it's his thick hair and dimples or his equanimity and confidence, but Ryan stands out in a crowd. Clean-cut, understated yet professional in his jeans, sports shirt and blue blazer, and successful yet humble, Ryan at first appeared reserved, but when I went up to talk with him, I found him warm and sincere. I remember thinking that, with his passion and creative ideas, he simply exudes happiness. I told him about my video project on happiness. "Would you be willing to be in it?" I asked. "Sure," Ryan said, shaking my hand and looking me right in the eyes, "I'd be glad to." He agreed to be filmed in my Minneapolis office.

Jenn: "Putting the truth out there connects you with more people."

I met Jenn when she and I appeared together in a performance piece called *The Naked I: Wide Open*, which presents original, locally written pieces on transgender experiences.

Tall and thin, Jenn nearly always wore a consignment-store tie and tweed driving cap. At first she seemed a bit awkward. Shy and reserved, she was harder to get to know than others in the cast. As we talked, I heard bits of her story—mental illness, bankruptcy. I was surprised because, despite all this, Jenn is someone who seems truly happy, and she said it is intentional. I wanted to know how she did that. Good news. She agreed to be interviewed on videotape. I brought my video camera and tripod to her funky Uptown Minneapolis apartment.

Tracy: "The thing that I like about my life now is I feel I have a purpose. There is something important for me to do that makes a difference."

My husband, Greg, nominated Tracy. He had known Tracy for more than 20 years.

"Tracy has always had a very independent spirit," Greg told me. "He follows his passions. He also happens to be tremendously talented, which maybe helps." Not necessarily, I think. You only have to grab the latest issue of *People Magazine* to read of the heartache of the talented. "I'd say it's his confidence," Greg continued. "He's just got this air of confidence. Not in a braggy way. He knows himself well. I've never known him to question what he likes or should do. He's just in it, and he does it." I'm intrigued. And I know there has to be more to the story. I added Tracy to the list. He's my eighth and final candidate. I was able to video him in his Chicago living room when I was there for a friend's wedding.

Now for the expert.

Henry Emmons, MD: "One of the long-standing sources of my real happiness is for me to be more and more fully who I am in every area of my life. I can't do psychiatry the way it has become any more. It took me a long time, but I am now able to be more completely myself in the work that I do. I don't just do medications. I just practice in a different way. I bring my undivided self to that work."

I learned about psychiatrist and author Henry Emmons, MD, long before I met him. Whenever my colleagues talked about Dr. Emmons, I heard an unmistakable reverence and awe in their voices.

I finally met him in person in the late 1990s. He was the consulting psychiatrist at a counseling center where I worked. Upon meeting him, it's easy to see what all the fuss was about. Smiling easily, Dr. Emmons seems calm and grounded. He's gentle and sincere. Appearing genuinely interested in others, he listens attentively. He seems very "real" and trustworthy. He is kind, compassionate, and egoless; in his presence, you feel that he truly appreciates you and what you have to say. That's not the only thing that sets Dr. Emmons apart. He is a rare psychiatrist in that he has studied both traditional Western medicines and alternative approaches, including nutritional supplements, Buddhist psychology, and Ayurvedic medicine. When he agreed to appear as my happiness "expert," I was overjoyed.

Granted, this list does not represent tremendous diversity. All are Caucasian and well educated. All but one work in a major metropolitan area. Two live in small towns. Ages range from mid-20s to early 60s. Some are single, some partnered, one divorced. Two subjects identify as women, five as men. One's gender identity is fluid. Some have children, some do not. Some are heterosexual, others not.

Needless to say, this isn't a scientific study. This is a personal quest. I want to know as much as I can about happiness, and these nine people seem to be the right ones to begin my journey with. I'm thrilled to share with you what I learned.

It's the day of filming, and my first four happiness interviewees finally arrive—Mia, Gretchen, Warren, and Dr. Emmons. To make the experience more personal (and to save money on renting a studio space), the initial filming is done at my Minneapolis home. Holding a list of 27 questions, I am well prepared. Here's a small sample:

- What is happiness to you?
- What brings meaning to your life? How important is that in your happiness?
- How do you overcome the hard times we all inevitably face?
- How do the important people in your life bring you happiness?
- How are you with taking risks?

I spent an entire day with joyful people hearing them talk about what makes them tick, and I have never been happier. There is something about talking about happiness that just makes you happy! Hands down, this day lives on as one of the best of my life.

On a break from filming, toward the end of the day, I step out on the back porch. As I savor the cool spring air and drink in the sight of the thick, newly grown green grass, I sigh. I am suffused with contentment. The depth of wisdom that comes from these interviews astounds me. If I am this happy from talking with happy people about their happiness, I think, it's probably true for others, as well. Wouldn't we all benefit from dialoguing with happy people, hearing what they do that makes them happy?

A moment later, I feel a jolt of electricity running down my spine as inspiration strikes. Continue the conversation about happiness, it says, and take it to as many people as you can. What my interviewees are telling me needs to be shared with a broader audience. I want to videotape more exceptionally happy people, write a book that covers the lessons I am learning, and share the profound experience of the process itself. There's magic in the very act of sitting with happy people and connecting deeply with them through talking about happiness.

In retrospect, I owe a debt of gratitude to my colleague. Had he not been so challenging, none of this likely would have happened. Under the right circumstances, of course, any of us is vulnerable to falling prey to a toxic co-worker, an abusive spouse, or a demoralizing friend. In my case, I realize the experience I had with my colleague triggered me into what Jungians call a "complex." A complex is an overwhelming, complicated psychological state with many connected parts, some of which are unknown to us. This state of being is complex—difficult to make sense of. In it, we are overwhelmed with thoughts and emotions and can't seem to find a way out on our own. I love this concept, as I find it so helpful with clients and in my own life in creating enough emotional distance to sort through difficult situations.

I realize now that on an unconscious level, trying desperately to appease a figure that was impossible to satisfy, my experiences with my coworker catapulted me into a complex. He reminded me of times in my life when I wasn't seen for who I truly am, including being bullied. Unable to avoid his caustic working style, I felt frustrated, helpless, and desperate—just as I felt when there was nothing I could do to prevent the earlier bullying.

I can see now that I gave my colleague way too much power. Part of me wishes I could have grounded myself more fully in the present, and realized that what was happening had nothing to do with me or my past, that his problems were not mine, and continued on with my work.

On the other hand, I can now say I'm glad it all happened. I never would have left my former dream job without the kind of motivation only deep misery provides. Without that prompt, I might not have returned to performing—certainly not when I did, and possibly not with the level of determination and commitment I ended up bringing to it. Returning to performing helped me realize a passion that had been dormant for decades and led me to deeply satisfying connections with people who are now close friends—people I now can't imagine living without. My reactions to my colleague helped me recognize how easily I still can become emotionally triggered when bullied (or when I am in a situation at all reminiscent of being bullied).

While I wouldn't wish such suffering on anyone, all my experiences—from cruel teenage classmates to a 20-something who created a hostile work environment—formed who I am. I've experienced everything from phenomenal joy, to paralyzing anxiety, to the depths of despair. Without the whole beautiful, catastrophic gestalt of it, I might not have been inspired to write this book.

CHAPTER 2

Defining happiness: Happiness explained?

What is this thing we call happiness? Its name comes from the Middle English word "hap," which means "good luck." Our ancestors appear to have believed that happiness favors only a fortunate few, and that there was little they could do to bring it about. Wellbeing was in the hands of fate, or the gods. While it's true that ancient wise men such as Plato, Socrates, and Aristotle believed we could earn happiness, the everyday person, toiling away just to survive, probably never found that to be so. And even to those sages, happiness came only after much effort. As Darrin M. McMahon, Ph.D., writes, "The ancients thought of happiness not as an emotional state but as an outcome of moral comportment."* Happiness was earned, then, by ethical behavior.

Fast forward a couple thousand years, and today's Merriam-Webster's online dictionary defines happiness as

a: a state of well-being and contentment: joy
b: a pleasurable or satisfying experience

So we have gone from viewing happiness as something that was predetermined by fate and then later earned by good deeds to today, where happiness is simply an experience of pleasure or joy based on our emotional state or a satisfying experience. That's a big leap in consciousness.

Small wonder that so many of us still fall back into believing the old idea that happiness is something that happens to us, rather than something we can make happen. For me, true happiness is much broader than the momentary pleasure implied by Merriam-Webster.

I was curious about how my interviewees, who seem happy so much of the time, would describe happiness. I asked each of them how they define happiness and how they know when they have attained it.

How does Warren know when he's truly happy? When comparing himself to unhappy folks, hairstylist Warren says, "I don't have any bitterness. I don't have many regrets." He looks philosophical. "I don't look back with remorse. I don't see any of that."

I understand what he's getting at. Happy people seem to live in the present. They don't dwell on the past or worry about the future. Those who aren't happy can't seem to get beyond their past, wishing they'd made different choices, or are consumed by how they were wronged.

In a similar vein, counseling center director Barry observes, "There are a lot of folks out there who feel like life is sort of crappy, and every once in a while you get a reprieve. I believe that everything is pretty darn fine, and every once in a while something terrible falls in. Which is just part of the tableau. And then things typically go back to okey dokey." I can't hold back a little giggle. Barry's glass-is-half-full philosophy is contagious. When I'm near him, I'm more optimistic, too. It's part of why I like him so much.

I ask Minneapolis therapist Mia how she knows she's happy. "I know I'm happy when things sort of flow in my life. I don't have to work too hard or push to make things happen. I think it also has a lot to do with my state of mind," she tells me, glancing down for a moment. "Not a lot of turning of the mind and thinking things over a lot. Just a sense of contentedness." With her warm smile and big heart, Mia is saying that when she's happy, she is in the moment. Life is flowing, and she's not ruminating.

When I'm down, I tend to spend a lot of time in my head replaying unpleasant memories, or worrying about what's to come. "Will that damn lawn ever get mowed?" I might ask myself. If I'm in a particularly prickly mood, I often predict negative outcomes. "Like usual, I'll probably have to do it myself," I can hear myself thinking. I might even sigh out loud, shake my head, and roll my eyes a bit. (Don't worry. While I know I can be dramatic, I make sure such movements are subtle in case anyone's watching.)

"I know I'm happy because I feel good," says Gretchen, the elegant singer and yoga teacher. "I feel this energy inside of me that makes me feel very alive, and I know that I'm growing and learning every day. And I'm really grateful. And that makes me feel very happy." Her feather earrings stir as she nods her head for emphasis. "I think that's what it means to be happy, is to be really grateful and present. And that's what I am."

Hmmm, so gratitude and being in the present are essential components in Gretchen's happiness. Yes, I realize! When I'm happier, I count my blessings more often. (At least I have a lawn to mow!) And Mia says almost the same thing. When she's happy, she's in the here and now. That's of course the present. (Okay. I'm not mowing the lawn now. Now I'm writing, which can be pretty darn fun.)

Relaxing in his workout clothes in his comfortable Chicago home, youth sports coach and fitness trainer Tracy tells me his understanding of the word has evolved. "In the past, happy to me would have been much more about laughing and jokes and having enough money. Creature comforts. Now," he explains, "My happiness has much more to do with peace and tranquility. And also the moments of what I would call unadulterated joy." And then he shares with me one of those moments:

"This morning, I was in a foul mood. I got about four hours of sleep," Tracy says, shaking his head. Walking to work on the sidewalk, wallowing, he was barely aware of his surroundings. His head down, he couldn't help but notice a message written in chalk at his feet. "Today thousands of small miracles will happen," he read.

His face begins to soften. "So I took a picture. And then I looked, and, oh my gosh, there's more. And I look, and the other one said, 'Today is an opportunity.'

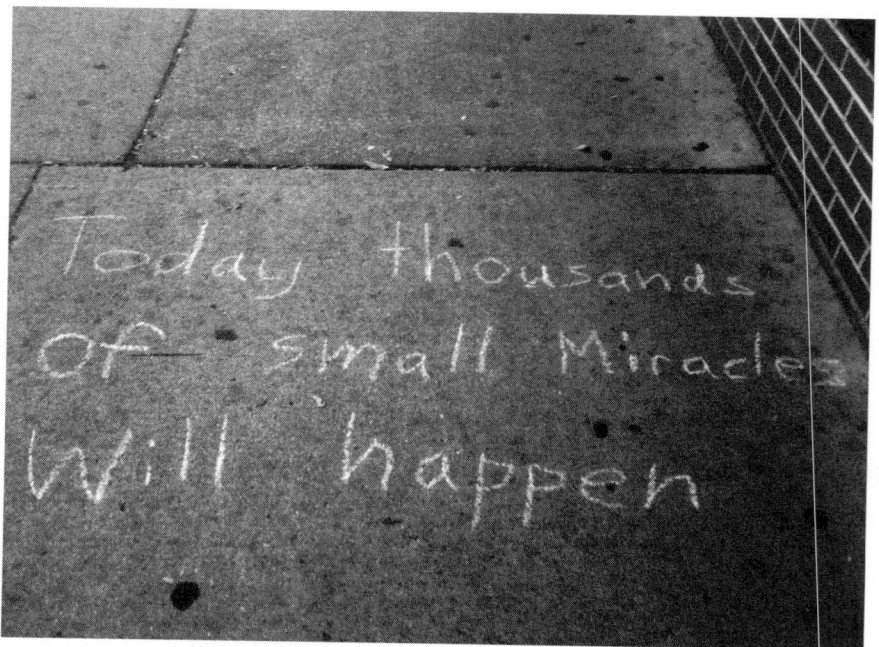

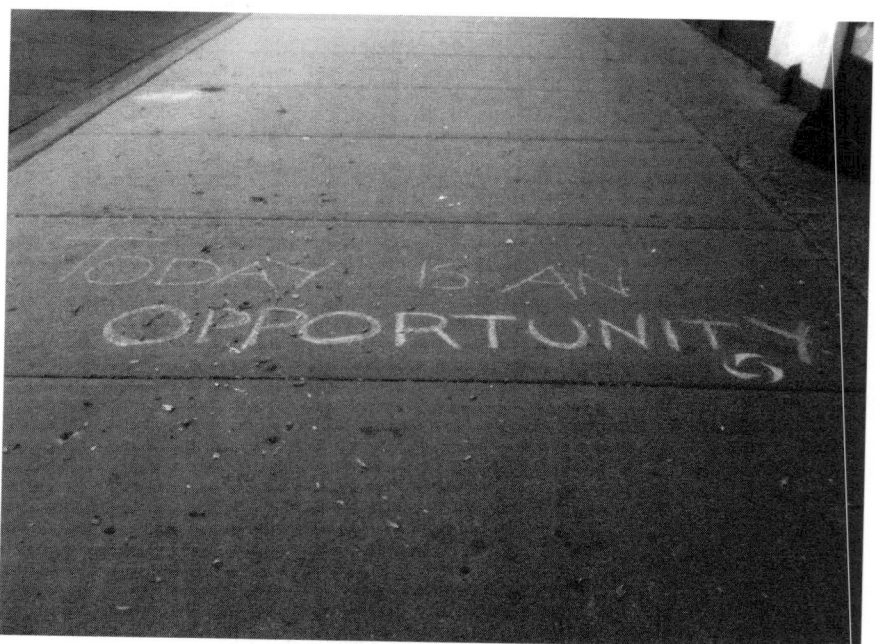

"Just reading these two things written on the sidewalk," Tracy gushes, "and my entire day was changed. Now I'm thinking, what's the opportunity today? To look at something as an opportunity as opposed to an obstacle. Instead of turmoil, you get peace and tranquility." Grinning fully now, Tracy is happy. So am I. Like laughter, happiness is contagious.

Are happy people always happy?

I interview Barry in his sunny Connecticut home. (I'd traveled out East to see my niece appear in a musical, and I was able to extend my long weekend trip to spend half a day with Barry.) With bright yet soothing colors adorning furniture and walls, and books spread on the coffee table between us, Barry's living room is as warm and colorful as he is. A stuffed bear watches from the corner. He's fixed us both tea, and as he leans back in his comfortable couch, I ask him if he's always happy. Barry tells me, "I'm not always happy. That seems unreasonable. Things upset me. It's okay to be upset about things that are upsetting. Bad things happen. Life is rife with terrible things. It's okay to be unhappy about unhappy things." But he doesn't stay there. "I have an unwavering belief that things tend to work out."

Philip feels the same. "Just because you're happy doesn't mean you're always smiling." All of us encounter bad times, this Detroit artist suggests. "Life is just ebbs and flows. They're a part of life." Accepting this helps him put harder times in perspective. "Bad things become inconsequential," he tells me, leaning forward. "It's the ability to see everything from 30,000 feet up," says Philip. Philip's happiness stems from embracing the good and the bad times, keeping perspective and maintaining faith.

Sitting next to a piano, her back straight, Gretchen tells me, "My definition of happiness is not necessarily joy, like smiles and laughter. I believe that is the result of happiness. I think real happiness is to be in a state of consciousness. To be very aware of the moment and taking it for what it is." (We'll talk more about awareness in Chapter 6: Developing mindfulness.)

One of my favorite formal happiness definitions comes from Matthieu Ricard, who holds a Ph.D. in molecular genetics. Ricard resigned from his promising yet unfulfilling scientific career to become a Buddhist monk. Years later, the press proclaimed him "The World's Happiest Man." In his book, *Happiness: A Guide to Developing Life's Most Important Skill*, Ricard defines happiness as, "a deep sense of flourishing that arises from an exceptionally healthy mind . . . an optimal state of being. Happiness is also a way of interpreting the world, since while it may be difficult to change the world, it is always possible to change the way we look at it."

Ricard continues: "Without inner peace and wisdom, *we have nothing we need to be happy.* Living on a pendulum between hope and doubt, excitement, and boredom, desire and weariness, it's easy to fritter away our lives, bit by bit, without even noticing, running all over the place and getting nowhere. Happiness is a state of inner fulfillment, not the gratification of inexhaustible desires for outward things."

Gretchen Rubin, whose book *The Happiness Project* is part of what inspired my own journey into exploring happiness, says she is asked often to define the term, but declines. On her website, she explains why. "A term can elude you as you try to define it." She goes on to point out that "one positive psychology study identified 15 different academic definitions of happiness." When it came to her own happiness project, however, she didn't find it helpful to distinguish between such terms as 'contentment,' 'positive affect,' 'subjective well-being,' and the like.

"I think it's enough to think about being 'happier,'" she says. "Even if we don't agree about what it means to be happy, we can agree that whatever happiness means, it would be nice to be happier. I think the looseness of the term happiness is actually helpful," she continues. "It's a concept large enough to embrace many different perspectives. I suspect that one reason people try to avoid using the word 'happiness' is that happiness has a bad reputation. It's often associated with superficiality, self-absorption, narcissism, and pleasure-seeking."

Who can blame folks for wanting to avoid association with such qualities? The truth, however, is that happier people are anything but selfish. As Rubin says, "Studies show that happiness doesn't make people complacent or self-centered. Rather, happier people are more likely to volunteer, to give away money, to persist in problem-solving, to help others, and to be friendly." People who define themselves as happy, in short, are more giving and contribute more to the world. Sounds like something worth pursuing to me!

Back to the question of definition, Rubin sums it up with this: "I know when I feel happy. Trying to be happier–that's good enough for me, without a precise definition."

I love the freedom this idea provides. Happiness is subjective; what happiness is to you may not be what happiness is to me. Whether you and I can agree on what it means doesn't not matter as much as the effect of our both working to become happier. The process of our working toward it may help us become better people who contribute more to the greater good—even if we're working on very different things.

I still think it is a helpful exercise, however, to define happiness for ourselves. After all, as the saying goes, if we don't know where we're going, we'll probably end up someplace else.

So what is happiness to *you*? Although just about everyone says they want to be happy, I find most people are stumped when asked to define the term. Creating a personal definition, in fact, is the initial assignment in my happiness classes. I suggest students start with images, because visual symbols and pictures access more of the brain than words alone. I bring in as many magazines as I can carry and ask my students to cut out (or draw, if they prefer) depictions and representations of what happiness means to them.

Before embarking on this video and writing journey, I wanted to be happy, but, like most people, didn't think much about what that truly meant. At the time, I viewed happiness as a state of being to strive for, and one that takes effort to attain. Although I was barely aware of this, I thought happiness was a destination—an emotional state we could arrive at and sustain. As I would find out, that definition would change radically.

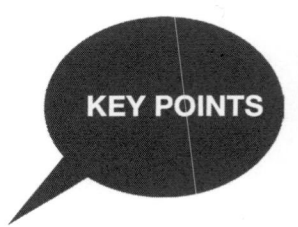

KEY POINTS

- Happiness doesn't mean always smiling or perpetually feeling good
- Happy people get down but don't stay stuck
- Maintaining perspective is key; happy people avoid getting mired down in minutia, and focus on what is truly important
- Awareness of the present moment breeds happiness
- Viewing difficulties as opportunities instead of obstacles provides perspective
- Establishing a common definition of this subjective term is challenging
- The process of becoming happier may be more important than being happy

PUTTING IT INTO PRACTICE

DEFINE Create your own definition of happiness. Most of us claim we want it but are hard pressed to say what happiness is to us.

1. Before using words, start with images. Cut out magazine pictures or printed web images that represent happiness to you. Try to get out of your mind—let the subconscious guide you. What images are you drawn to? If you want, draw images that make you feel happy. Allow yourself to draw or cut out more images than you might eventually use.
2. Get a large piece of paper or poster board.
3. Once you've got a large pile or number of images, place them all out in front of you. What themes or patterns emerge?

COLLATE Using the images above, create a happiness collage. Make it as utilitarian or beautiful as you wish. Glue the images to your paper or poster board.

DRAFT Now that you've got images in front of you to engage both sides of the brain, begin to find words to express your unique definition of happiness. Perhaps use prompts like this to get you going:
- I know I'm happy when . . .
- To me, happiness is . . .
- When happy, my body feels . . .
- I'm happiest when I'm doing . . .

_____

_____

_____

_____

_____

_____

Let this list sit for a few hours or a few days. Continue to revise or rewrite it as you like. It may take several drafts before you identify the themes that point to what happiness truly is to you. Likewise, in the days following completion of your collage, you may come across additional images. Allow it to be a work in progress.

_____

_____

_____

_____

_____

_____

MONITOR For a week or so, track your happiness throughout the day. Note what you are doing when you are happiest. Carry a notebook, or use the notepad feature on your smartphone. You might try websites and/or apps such as TrackYourHappiness.org.

WHAT THEMES DO YOU NOTICE?

_____

_____

_____

_____

_____

_____

WHEN ARE YOU THE LOWEST? WHAT ARE YOU DOING?

_____

_____

_____

_____

_____

_____

*Darrin McMahon: http://www.yesmagazine.org/happiness/a-history-of-happiness

CHAPTER 3

Finding your happiness set-point: The coffee table syndrome

I met Kanesha at a professional training conference almost 25 years ago, but her story about happiness has stayed with me. On a coffee break during that first workshop, Kanesha told me how she once had been convinced that she would be truly happy when she obtained the one item missing from her downtown St. Paul apartment: a leather couch. After saving for months, Kanesha—with great joy—finally ordered her coveted sofa. When a large truck pulled up outside her apartment, she could barely keep herself from jumping up and down. Her long-awaited brown leather couch at last had arrived! She gave the deliverymen specific instructions as to where to place the couch so that it would be just so—a hand's width from the wall, facing the TV, centered under the living room window. Always highly expressive, Kanesha demonstrated with sweeping, staccato hand motions.

During those first few days, Kanesha said she found herself glorying in fondness for and appreciation of her new acquisition. She could hardly wait to get home from work each night so she could sprawl across her new, comfy prize. It was just what she'd wanted and worked so hard for. "Yeah," she told me, her head shaking slightly, "that happiness lasted maybe a week—until I realized I didn't have the right coffee table." Out of the corner of my eye, I saw that the volume of Kanesha's resulting laughter caused those nearby to momentarily pause and stare. Kanesha didn't seem to notice (or to care if she did). I just shook my head in delight at this big-hearted new friend with a story to which we all can relate.

In my case, it wasn't a couch. It was money—as in a particular level of income. I was convinced that if I just made a certain amount of money, I would be happy. I was in my late 20s at the time, and the economy had tanked. With it went my fulltime job. To pay rent and put food on the table, I had to juggle three part-time jobs: employee assistance counselor, childcare worker, and restaurant server. Still barely making enough to get by, I discovered clever ways to cut expenses. To avoid paying for parking meters or ramps, I became a master at finding free on-street parking spaces. When I was able to afford to see a movie, I bought a pack of gum from the corner drug store first instead of the pricey concession-stand popcorn. Rather than joining a gym (which I longed to do), I took long walks around the city, even in the bitter winter chill. I avoided seeing a doctor or dentist until the last possible moment.

I was convinced that all my worries would be behind me once I made a particular annual salary. With time and effort, thankfully, I did reach that income level. In some ways, life indeed became easier. I joined the gym I wanted, visited medical professionals as needed, and didn't have to skip the popcorn at the movie theater. Looking back, I realize that while I was less stressed about sheer survival after I hit my income level goal, new worries quickly replaced the old ones. Now, in order to be happy, I "needed" a tape deck for my car. My new workplace went through a major reorganization, turning my work life upside down. I was single and desperately longed to have a partner. Slowly, it began to dawn on me that although my paycheck went up, my overall happiness level didn't change.

Who hasn't experienced something similar? It can be oh so tempting to believe that the right sweater or vacation or job or degree is all we'll need to make us happy. But once we obtain that sought-after goal, soon enough the shine fades, and like Kanesha, we're right back where we started—looking for that certain something missing that is sure to make us happy. I call this "The Coffee Table Syndrome." My clients know the story all too well.

Psychologists often use such cases to illustrate the theory that we each have a particular "set-point" of happiness. In common language, "set-point" is sometimes used to signify an individual's "constitution," or even "personality." Whatever it's called, the implication is that, much like our personality, one's set-point cannot vary. The idea is that at birth we inherit a certain level of happiness, and that is all we are going to get because the set-point is inflexible. This old concept seems to be employed most frequently by those who are less than happy and who feel there is nothing they can do about it. We are born with a certain happiness capacity level, and that's all there is to it.

The set-point theory came into vogue in a 1971 essay entitled, "Hedonic Relativism and Planning the Good Society," by P. D. Brickman and Donald T. Campbell, published in *Adaptation Level Theory: A Symposium* (New York: Academic Press, 1971). Psychologists Brickman and Campbell observed that regardless of whether they encounter an unhappy setback or a very happy event, in due time people nearly always return to their innate set-point of happiness.

According to the set-point theory, after "recovering" from a good or bad event, we tend to return to our genetic set-point, or our average daily mood, which was determined at birth. Those who already lean toward being positive or optimistic, then, tend to return to that state no matter how rough (or blissful) a particular time may be. Likewise, those with more pessimistic outlooks tend to experience the same return to their "grumpy old selves," even after experiencing some kind of windfall.

While there is no doubt this phenomenon exists, not everyone is convinced that that's all there is to it. Psychologist Robert Biswas-Diener, for instance, says happiness is much more nuanced. Biswas-Diener (who, thanks to his international travel exploring happiness, is sometimes called the "Indiana Jones of positive psychology") says, "The formula for happiness for any individual is derived from a unique synergy of genetics, environment, and behavior." Therefore it is absurd, he contends, to claim that an individual's happiness is due to any one factor, including his or her innate set-point. The set-point theory, then, at least according to this Harrison Ford of the psychology world, is far too simple for beings as complex as we humans.

Even if we acknowledge that genetics may be part of the happiness formula, it is only one player. What else is involved, and how much of a role do these various factors play? Psychologist Sonja Lyubormirsky tackled these questions in her book, *The How of Happiness*.

Lyubormirsky found that genetics do, indeed, influence one's happiness level. But circumstances or situations also affect it. These are sometimes called "environmental factors." Examples of circumstances that can shape our happiness include education, race, gender, age, career, marital status, and religion. Family of origin, health, relationships, and income also play a part in our situation and circumstances.

How much of an impact do genetic and environmental factors have on our happiness? Take a guess. What portion of your happiness would you say is governed by genetic factors (aka set-point)? Eighty or 90 percent? Actually, Lyubormirsky found that only about 50 percent of our happiness (or unhappiness) level is "set," according to our genes.

So if half our happiness comes from nature, how much comes from environmental factors? Would you say the other 50 percent? According to Lyubormirsky, circumstances and situational factors together account for a measly, puny, tiny 10 percent.

Adding internal and external factors together, it would seem that 60 percent of our happiness comes from our set-point and environment. While it may be true that our happiness set-point cannot be moved very much, and we can't alter some circumstances such as our past or our family of origin, Lyubormirsky says this "doesn't mean that your happiness level cannot be changed."

If we do the happiness math, we're provided a 40 percent portion that we can influence. This 40 percent is what Lyubormirsky refers to as "intentional activity," or what I call "deliberate choices," and that's what much of this book explores.

Happily, new scientific discoveries are proving that genes aren't so fixed after all. As happiness expert Dr. Henry Emmons explains in his video interview with me, "Genetics do not create an unchangeable condition. Genetic expression can vary based upon circumstances." Dr. Emmons is referring to epigenetics. This relatively new science—one that was entirely new to me at the time—explains that while we may possess certain specific genes, those genes don't automatically become active; they could just as easily remain dormant. In other words, genes can get turned on or can remain in the off position. All sorts of factors, such as diet, environment, physical activity levels, and stress, can cause gene activation. "So our DNA may not vary," says Dr. Emmons, "but the way that DNA gets expressed changes depending upon circumstances. So even something like an emotional set-point is changeable, as it turns out."

Dr. Emmons explains that it is possible to change the ways your brain is hardwired. "It is possible, through doing things like mindfulness practice, to actually change your brain in ways. You can grow your frontal lobes, especially the healthy part of the frontal lobes. You can create a greater sense of openness and awareness. Your emotional set-point can be changed through consciousness practices. It's not as stable and stuck as we used to think." This is happy news indeed.

As I interviewed the happiest people I know, I realized that while they all seem to have a high happiness set-point, their external factors were wildly diverse. What they all have in common is a deep intentionality. They are all aware that their daily choices can make enormous contributions to their happiness level.

In the chapters ahead, we'll explore the choices these happiness makers make. Why do they do it, and how?

CHAPTER 4

Establishing a foundation: The self-care investment

My graduate school advisor, Dr. Brandt, was the first to point out a mysterious pattern to me. "Why do you think you're getting so many colds?" Dr. Brandt knew I had been to the campus health center a month earlier, only to be told there was nothing wrong, just one cold after another.

"Germs," I say with a shrug. Dr. Brandt's expressionless face makes me even more nervous than usual in her stern presence. "Living on campus," I stumble on, unable to hide the nasal sound made by my stuffed nose, "I'm swimming in a sea of germs."

"If that's the case, then why isn't everyone sick?" she asks.

Good question, even if I was too congested to think about it. With the help of liberal doses of Kleenex and throat lozenges, I was somehow able to focus enough to make it through the meeting. But Dr. Brandt's question stayed with me. I started to notice that after particularly stressful periods at school, I inevitably came down with a cold or sinus infection. If minor upper respiratory infections are caused solely by exposure to germs, then why weren't my classmates coming down with an equal number of colds and sinus infections? Here I was learning tremendous amounts of psychological theory and practice, but I had yet to read anything on the connection between stress and illness, let alone how to take care of oneself. The idea of "self-care" wasn't even on the radar in my graduate courses.

Even today, finding a good definition of self-care is harder than one might expect. Many I found were part of college or university health center websites. North Carolina State University defines self-care as "active participation in enhancing the quality of your health." University of Kentucky considers self-care "any intentional actions you take to care for your physical, mental and emotional health." The World Health Organization says, "Self-Care is the ability of individuals, families and communities to promote health, prevent disease, and maintain health and to cope with illness and disability with or without the support of a health-care provider."*

My definition of self-care? Reducing or eliminating undue stress, attending to physical needs (rest, wholesome foods, physical activity), creating an external environment that is soothing and centering, and maintaining relationships that provide emotional support. Perhaps better still is the definition of extreme self-care created by the pioneer in the modern personal coaching movement, Thomas Leonard: "Going to great lengths to show affection and concern for oneself." Now there's a concept. We go to great lengths for our loved ones; why not extend the same level of attention to ourselves?

I was intrigued when I learned how important self-care was to my interviewees. Was self-care a key component in their happiness? I also wanted to know how long they had they been actively practicing self-care, because I was beginning to think that the more constant your self-care, the more constant your happiness.

Nearly all my interviewees are physically active on a daily basis. One swims. Two take long walks. Another two practice yoga. Three of my interviewees are serious athletes—one rides his bicycle religiously, another has recently taken up rock climbing, and the third runs marathons.

We Need to Move

As Dr. Emmons settles into his upholstered chair for his video interview, I am struck by how peaceful and even-keeled he appears. While he's clearly brilliant, he remains approachable and humble. He is also calm—seemingly unflappable—and his pleasant, easy-going nature feels palpable. Even his shirt is a reassuring shade of light green. One of the first things I ask him is, "What simple, straightforward things can anyone do to be happier?"

"Our bodies need to move," he replies without a pause. "We have to recognize that we were not meant to be sedentary," says Dr. Emmons emphatically. "A hundred years ago, almost nobody was sedentary. Almost everybody worked on a farm or in agriculture, or somehow worked with their bodies," he tells me. "And we just have to remember we need to move, to get warmed up, to get sweaty. It doesn't have to be anything fancy. Walking, it turns out, is a really great activity for boosting mood. Really good," he emphasizes.

Walking improves our moods? How can the simple act of walking impact our brain and our perception of how we are feeling? Isn't that all based on what is going on in our lives at any given point? Would a 20-minute walk really help someone who just got disappointing news?

According to Dr. Emmons, it probably would. Most physical activities trigger the release of endorphins, he explains. Endorphins activate the opiate receptors in the brain, reducing the perception of pain and suffering of all kinds—physical as well as emotional. In fact, endorphins have a similar effect on the brain as certain drugs like morphine and codeine. A daily 20- to 30-minute walk can improve sleep and increase mental acuity when awake, Dr. Emmons continues. Calming the emotional centers in the brain and nervous system, walking reduces stress.

While many claim they're too tired to exercise or fear that movement will deplete them, walking actually increases energy levels, Dr. Emmons tells me. How often do you feel invigorated after a walk with a friend or with your dog?

"Biking is part of the foundation that keeps me happy"

"Biking makes me very happy," hairstylist Warren tells me during our Minneapolis video interview. "Biking is part of the foundation that keeps me happy and keeps everything in my life in balance. I spend a lot of time on the bike. I ride a couple hundred miles a week at least." His lean frame, clear complexion, and quick wit make the claim plausible. A contagious smile covers his face. "When people ask me, 'Why do you bike so much?' I joke and say, 'So I don't come home and chop my family up into little pieces.'" Warren chuckles. "I'm joking of course. What it really does is it sets me right. It's meditative," Warren offers, a look of serenity settling on his features. "Biking brings me a lot of joy," Warren continues. "I am so at peace on the bicycle. I do it in the rain. I'll do it in the snow. I'll do it in my basement on a stationary bike. I do it anywhere. Ask anyone. They'll tell ya, 'He's on a bike. If he's not here, he's gone biking.'"

Wow, I think. That's quite a testament. Warren's consistent self-care in the form of physical activity both soothes and brings him joy. What impressed me was how his biking was so deeply a part of his identity; clearly, he had been biking intensely for years.

"It's life changing"

Another interviewee, the clean-cut Minneapolis filmmaker Ryan, is also an avid bicyclist—and he's on the same page as Warren: "I think physical activity is huge. I don't know what I'd do without it. It's a big reason why I ride my bike everywhere. I have to be well enough to ride my bike just to travel for transportation. I have to stay in shape just for that," he says. "Plus, it just makes me feel good," he adds.

He also recently took up rock climbing and is quick to extoll its multiple benefits. "It's almost life changing," Ryan gushes. "When you're out there climbing, you can't think about anything else, because when you do, that's when you're going to fall off. Having that physical activity where you are concentrating 100 percent, you can block everything out. If there are things stressing you out or weighing you down," Ryan continues, his face serious, "you can get rid of it for a short period of time. And then when you're done climbing, you have that sense of euphoria from just being physically active."

Ryan is pointing out physical activity's double virtue: The required focus clears his mind, acting as a powerful stress reducer. As for the euphoria Ryan mentions, that's the aforementioned endorphins at work.

Like all of us, I had heard for years that we need to exercise to be healthy, but I never truly understood why and how. Simply being told "exercise and a nutritious diet are good for you" started sounding like a typical mother's tired refrain, "because I said so." It didn't work when I was small, and admonishments like that don't work now that I have grown.

What did work was gaining a fuller comprehension of how exercise actually works. For me, author Chris Crowley provided that understanding. His was the first self-help book that I read on exercise that actually made sense to me. In his book, *Younger Next Year*, he and his co-author Dr. Henry Lodge explain how stress impacts our bodies. Their down-to-earth tone makes the intricate science of exercise and nutrition suddenly clear and understandable.

As the authors explain, our bodies contain master chemicals called cytokines. Cytokines are small proteins that reside in many of the cells that course through our blood, and their job is to signal cells to act in certain ways. Crowley and Lodge describe two different types of cytokines: Cytokine-6 (or C-6), which cause inflammation of cells and their eventual decay, and Cytokine-10 (or C-10), which prompt cells to repair and grow.

C-6 and C-10 are intimately entwined. When we are young, we have a lot of C-10 cytokines coursing through our blood that tell us to grow, grow, grow. As we enter our 30s, however, our bodies are programmed to begin a steady release of C-6 cytokines. These trigger cellular inflammation, which eventually leads to cellular death. This is nature's way of making us age.

Inflammation is damage caused for the most part by stress—only it's inside our bodies, so we can't see it. Well, what if you could see it? What do you imagine internal inflammation looks like? In my mind, I see otherwise ordinary-looking amoeba things, only their tips are red, with puss-filled, crusty white edges. Not pretty, I know. But the nastier you get with this visualization the better. With portions damaged, your body must work harder than necessary to repair itself, further taxing an already overwrought system. I realize now that this is precisely why I was getting sick so often in grad school.

Nature, however, provides a brilliant little safety valve. If you get a huge blast of C-6, say from the stress of being threatened by a tiger and fleeing for your life, that excess C-6 will trigger the release of C-10, which in turn mops up all that nasty C-6 that results in decay and aging. The net result is less decay, less aging. Moving our bodies stimulates an elegant system of repair and growth. Moreover, if you get a daily dose of C-10, you can literally halt that decay process of C-6 and ensure a daily dose of growth and repair.

Chronic stress is just as bad as acute stress

In *Younger Next Year,* Crowley writes, "With the chronic stress of modern life, the chemistry of inflammation persists but the renovation never gets started. Decay becomes a career path for your body, and your blood itself becomes an inflammatory, caustic stew of C-6, carrying decay throughout. Not chronic stress as in two months of drought or four months of winter, but chronic stress as in decades of emotional strain, decades of being sedentary and overweight, decades of living in isolation. The tide is set against you." Why? Because C-6 does not always trigger the production of C-10. "When sedentary, there is a steady, slow drip of inflammation, but not enough to turn on C-10. That explosion of growth comes only with the surge of C-6 you get with exercise." This is particularly true with active, strenuous aerobic activity. The cure has always been right in front of us: serious aerobic exercise. Because it produces a large amount of C-10, aerobic activity triggers repair, renewal, and growth.

"Chronic emotional stress also produces a trickle of background C-6," Crowley says. "[With daily exercise,] at least enough to sweat, not only are you guaranteed to be fit, you'll be healthy, more relaxed, more optimistic. Why? Because C-10 will automatically flood your body an hour after exercise like a sprinkler coming on at sundown." This rush of C-10 restores what you lost from all the C-6 that was released from sitting around all day. Furthermore, it's not just stress and disease that can trigger ill health. "Loneliness, apathy, too much alcohol and TV all trigger the inflammatory part of the cycle," Crowley continues. Exercise, commitment to caring relationships and meaningful work, and having fun provide the antidote. Crowley may not have set out to write a book about happiness, but his program of exercise, eating right, and maintaining caring relationships surely promotes it.

If I had known in graduate school that the cure for my colds was exercise, I'm not sure I would have believed it. In junior high and high school, I would have been considered an "anti-athlete." Those popular "jock" types were often the ones who bullied me, yelling "queer" at me in crowded hallways between classes, writing "fag" on my locker. My adolescent mind associated people who exercise with cruelty. Breaking a sweat, I unconsciously believed, would be betraying myself. Turns out I was to have the last laugh; despite my abhorrence for athletes, I was always drawn to running. Seeing runners propel their bodies forward looked like fun, and I admired the focus and serenity in runners' gazes as they stride. It was the early 1980s, and the running craze was in full swing. Immediately following my high school graduation—the very next day, no less—I went for my first run. Not wanting anyone to see me (would I look prissy? Would my cheeks puff out and eyes bulge? Would I collapse from over exertion?), I waited until it was pitch dark before setting out.

I expected I'd be drained after running, but I wasn't exhausted afterward. I actually had *more* energy! And I enjoyed it. I felt good physically and mentally. I was proud that I'd accomplished something for my health. Within a few short weeks, my confidence buoyed, I no longer feared looking ridiculous. I decided it was time to run in the daytime. (Daylight, of course, offered the additional benefit of helping me avoid potholes and other hazards.)

Thirty-plus years later, running is still my preferred exercise. Running comes naturally to me, and while it takes effort, it doesn't seem like work. I feel free when I run, and yes, happy. When I don't run, I feel cranky, negative, and irritable. In brutal Midwest winters, I run on our basement treadmill or bundle up and take the dog for long, quiet walks near an ice-covered lake. I also do strength training a few times a week, including squats, pushups, kettle bell swings, ab roller, and a strength band. But inevitably, the first sign of spring brings an urge to run that I can barely control. Whenever I see other runners peacefully pounding the pavement, a sense of envy overcomes me. How satisfying it is to attend high school reunions, where I am now far more fit than the former athletes who bullied me!

Thanks to Crowley's book, I now understand why running makes me feel the way it does. In fact, I have come to see exercise in a whole new light. An hour or so after a good workout, it's as though I can feel the chemical rush streaming through my body, as though my insides are being saturated in a bath of soothing, rejuvenating, reparative soup. Those amoebas with the red tips and puss-filled, crusty white edges? They are healed in the bath created by exercise, rest, and healthier foods. Instead of being red and crusty (in my imagination), they're now a uniform, attractive shade of pink, with smooth edges.

We are what we eat

Crowley and Lodge also cover the importance of eating healthy foods. They say eating lean proteins and lots of vegetables and avoiding processed foods and refined sugars produces C-10. So does getting sufficient sleep and rest. Remember, C-10s fight inflammation, and detoxify and repair the body and mind.

When I eat a salad with a lean protein for lunch, I don't have that mid-afternoon slump I tend to get after a sandwich, chips, and a cookie. Crowley's book got me wondering, how important is nutrition to happiness? I wanted to see if my interviewees believe food choices impact their happiness.

"My body feels better"

During our interview, I ask Jenn about the importance of nutrition in her happiness. "I try not to put too much sugar in my body," she tells me. Living a half block from the Wedge Natural Foods Cooperative near downtown Minneapolis, a wide selection of wholesome is steps from her door. Jenn does "wise shopping" at the Wedge, choosing whole foods—fresh fruits and vegetables, lean proteins and whole grains, all organic and local whenever possible. "We eat healthy, and my body feels better."

Also, stopping drinking alcohol was huge for Jenn. "That's another contributing factor to my happiness," she notes, "ridding those things of my body that aren't allowing me to be in the present moment." Here Jenn makes a significant point. In the long run, alcohol and other drugs dull our senses, taking us out of the present moment. Cloudier perceptions and experiences make it harder to appreciate the richness of what's right in front of us. Clarity of mind and purpose, conversely, return us to the fullness of what's happening right now. As Jenn says, "I have so much more clarity, and I'm much more present." Being more fully in this moment increases the opportunity to be satisfied and happy. (More on this in Chapter 6: Developing mindfulness.)

I have come to believe that eating well, limiting alcohol and other recreational drug intake, and getting adequate physical activity provide a foundation in which happiness becomes possible. By itself, it's not sufficient to create happiness, mind you, but good self-care establishes the base from which happiness may flourish.

"I try to eat well," says Philip, the hoodie-wearing Detroit artist, during his happiness video. "I'm big on eating vegetables, leafy greens." Why vegetables? "Because I feel better when I do," he says with a shrug. "I'm happier." It's important to note that it can take a while to notice a difference in mood from eating. It seems the effects may be cumulative, and it takes time for the body to flush itself of residual less-healthy foods. Some say, for example, that it takes about a month for sugar to be cleared from the system.

SNORES AND SNORTS

Another key component in self-care is sleep. According to a report from the Centers for Disease Control and Prevention, almost one-third of US working adults get six or fewer hours of sleep each night. For years, I was one of those adults. Thank goodness my partner, Greg, was so fed up with my snoring that he all but forced me to get a sleep study. Turns out I have sleep apnea. Until then, I thought everyone woke up several times each night; I thought it was normal. And I had no clue that it was my own snoring that was waking me. I've come to realize what a large role lack of sleep played in my coming down with colds and other upper-respiratory ailments during and beyond graduate school. Unsexy as it is, I now sleep much more soundly with a C-PAP (breathing machine).

THE IMPORTANCE OF SETTING INTENTION

"What I put in my body really matters," Minneapolis psychotherapist Mia tells me during our filmed interview. It's clear that she really thinks seriously about this. "The thing I did right before I came here. I thought, 'Oh, I am going to this interview. I need to manifest happiness, and I know that's in me. So how am I going to do that?'"

Mia pauses and tilts her head slightly. "So I had a green smoothie—vegetables, all spun up together." She's sitting cross-legged on the couch nearby, her thick, blond hair luminescent in the rays of the midmorning sun streaming through the window. "I think about that a lot—the internal environment. You know, where's my intention and what sort of nourishment am I giving myself. Food nourishment."

It sounds so simple, but let's break this down. Mia's objective is to talk with me clearly and thoughtfully about happiness. Before meeting with me, she checked in with herself, asking what she could do to help bring about her desired outcome. What came to her was to support what she calls her "internal environment"—her body and mind—by feeding it healthfully. This led her to make a luscious vegetable smoothie brimming with vitamins and phytochemicals. Other components of Mia's self-care include daily meditation and yoga three or four times a week. These keep Mia's mind and body calmer and more nimble. In this state, she is more grounded in the present, flexible and adaptable, and has more access to the fullness of her resources. Being able to go with the flow, Mia tells me, is a fundamental aspect of her happiness. Attending to her "internal environment" with nutrition and activity enables her to go with the flow. She has been doing this for years.

In my work as a life coach and psychologist, I see how easy it is for my clients to be so consumed with their busy lives that they lose sight of why they're doing it all to begin with. As one of my old, favorite sayings goes, "If you don't know where you're going, you'll probably end up somewhere else." Living with intention helps us avoid the unconscious, mindless decisions we might later regret. Rather than going on autopilot, intention starts with clarifying our values. Keeping what is important to us in the forefront of our minds helps us make more conscious decisions and maintain self-discipline.

"Exercise and eating a healthier diet helps everyone," Dr. Emmons says with great conviction. I know he's studied nutrition copiously, and I suspect he eats well himself. He looks great. There's not an ounce of fat on him, his kind eyes are crystal clear, and his mind is sharp and quick.

"If we're paying attention," he continues, "it becomes pretty easy to see that food has an effect on our mood. What we eat within a half hour, forty-five minutes, is going to affect our cognition, the way we can focus and concentrate, the energy in the body, and very often also the mood. So choosing foods that are really right for our body. Noticing the things that make us feel kind of jittery or sluggish and doing our best to reduce those foods—that's a choice you make multiple times a day."

I asked for specific examples.

"Sugar and caffeine are the things that can be over-stimulating for people's moods and bodies," he says. "I would say sugar really has a big impact on mood and on long-term health. Not just sugar, but simple carbs that quickly get converted into blood sugar impact the brain and really the rest of the body, creating inflammation and problems with insulin. We're just not meant to have that much simple carbohydrate. It's just not how our bodies evolved."

"So you're promoting whole grains?" I ask.

Dr. Emmons nods and looks to the side for a split second. It doesn't take him long to gather his thoughts. "The types of foods that I think are most helpful in keeping blood sugar stable and therefore affecting mood," he continues, "fall into three categories: whole grains, root vegetables, and beans and legumes." He suggests we eat "a lot of those foods with every meal," along with "protein and a few healthy fats."

What does he consider to be healthy fats? "One of the biggest changes in our diets in the last hundred years is that we do not get anywhere near as much Omega-3s as our ancestors did," Dr. Emmons tells me, nodding. "That makes a very big difference in mood, because it changes the way the brain works, and it can promote inflammation. The real problem is that we get way too much Omega-6 compared to Omega-3. They're both healthy, it turns out, but not when the ratio is so skewed. So the best thing we can do is add more Omega-3s to our diet."

Omega-3 and Omega-6 are types of essential fatty acids. Here, "essential" means we cannot make them on our own, so we must obtain them from our diet. But it can be handy to recall another meaning of the word "essential," as Omega-3s and Omega-6s are vital for obtaining and sustaining optimum health. According to the University of Maryland Medical Center, Omega-6 fatty acids play a crucial role in brain function, as well as in normal growth and development. Omega-3 fatty acids reduce inflammation and may help lower risk of chronic diseases.

Refined vegetable oils (such as corn, safflower, sunflower, and soy), many salad dressings and mayonnaise, most fast and packaged or refined foods, and even some nuts and seeds (brazil nuts, pumpkin seeds, walnuts, pine nuts, almonds, sesame seeds, pecans, and peanuts) contain large amounts of Omega-6s.

"Where can we find Omega-3s?" I inquire.

"Seafood, nuts, some seeds like hemp, chia, and flax," Dr. Emmons tells me. "Those are all good sources of Omega-3s. Olive oil is a good source. And I think for most people, it's a good idea to take some fish oil or some kind of Omega-3 supplement."

What we put in our body today pays off in the brain we have in a year

I am beginning to see that it is the daily intention to be happy that allows people to do the next right thing. Over time, these intentions become habits. Dr. Emmons sheds light on why these foundational pieces are so important long-term. "This moment is the result of all the moments that came before," he tells me, his voice resonant and calm. "What we do today is an investment in the brain and the body that we have six months or a year from now. Exercise makes most people feel good right away, but it is also going to add benefits months and years down the road. Same with diet. It becomes part of the body, and it's going to have healthful effects for years down the road."

Dr. Emmons adds, "I do a lot of work with people with depression, of course, in my work as a psychiatrist." His face appears serious. "The research on exercise as an effective treatment for depression is really compelling. It is a more effective intervention than medication. Most people consider medications to be the most powerful treatment of depression, but if you really look at the research, exercise works better, especially in the long run. Our bodies are simply meant to move." Dr. Emmons happened to have been on hand when I interviewed Warren, and he was clearly struck by what he heard. "Warren talked about biking and how important that was to him," Dr. Emmons recalls. "The way he phrased it, how biking spares his family because it helps him stay calm and steady. I just think that exercise can be as effective as medications for treating depression."

I'm sure Dr. Emmons doesn't mean to disparage antidepressants. They have their place. He is pointing out, however, that physical activity can be even more helpful. Study after study confirms that exercise improves mood. In a meta-analysis, investigators at the University of Toronto analyzed more than 26 years of research and concluded that even moderate activities, such as walking 20–30 minutes a day, wards off depression for people of all ages.**

If exercise even helps folks with clinical depression, imagine how it can help the rest of us feel happier. I had to know if Dr. Emmons practices what he preaches.

"I do practice what I preach," he tells me, smiling. "I'm not saying that I'm excellent at it," he admits, his head tilting slightly. "But I do practice it. I eat well. I exercise. Well, I should say I eat well most of the time. And I find that giving ourselves a break now and then, not being too rigid about doing everything right—at least for me—that's helpful."

Here, I think we need to go back to Mia's idea about intention. If we're eating mindlessly, then our attention is elsewhere, and we barely taste what's in our mouth. On the other hand, indulging every now and again in a favorite food, truly savoring each mouthful, now that's helpful. It's when we open the door to mindless eating that we get into trouble. (You'll find far more on the concept of mindfulness in Chapter 6: Developing mindfulness.)

"I USED TO DO SO MANY THINGS I HATED": THE STORY OF JACK

After working on self-care for a year, a client had a happiness epiphany: "I'm consuming far less alcohol, I eat better, and I exercise almost every day," Jack told me. "Taking one step at a time also helped me make these changes stick. As an engineer, I wish it could be simple, that X leads to Y and on to Z, but I appreciate now that human change is more complicated. There's no silver bullet. I used to do so many things I hated. My intention going forward is to continue to do things that make me happy."

Focus on Immediate Benefits

I asked my interviewees how important exercise and food is to them. A standout response came from Chicago fitness trainer Tracy, who emailed me: "I do definitely believe that good nutrition and exercise can lead to a greater sense of well-being and, most likely, more happiness." He says the fitness industry has it all wrong when they emphasize long-term health benefits as the reason people should work out. We've been told for years to get off our asses, yet Americans continue to get fatter. "We unfortunately view exercise as work leading to other things, such as losing weight, disease prevention, etc." Tracy writes. What actually motivates people to stick with exercise, however, is focusing on the immediate benefits. Tracy's own routine provides a good example. Echoing Warren, "I still go on a daily walk in the morning," and like Warren he jokingly adds that his daily walk is what makes him suitable "for contact with other humans."

I learned first hand about focusing on the immediate gain when I tried to exercise to lose weight for an upcoming high school reunion. "I'm going to eat really well and exercise every day for the next six months," I told myself, thinking my lean and thinner form would impress my former classmates. Those resolutions lasted maybe a week.

I've since become convinced that these new habits didn't take hold because I was undertaking them for the wrong reason—trying to "wow" others instead of caring for myself. It was like a holdover from those insecure adolescent days, believing I wasn't good enough just as I am. Coming from a place of self-doubt instead of self-love undermines our best intentions.

The importance of loving self-care finally became apparent last summer. While rehearsing and performing for months in the musical Hello, Dolly!, I dropped that five pounds without even trying. Though every dance rehearsal and each performance was like a marathon, I was dancing for the pure joy of it. When you have a simple, positive, unselfish goal in mind—such as joyful dancing—good things align. Unlike prepping for my reunion, this time I started from a place of self-love. I was doing an activity I'm wild about for the sheer joy of the activity itself, with the aim of sharing that joy with others. Engaging in activities we are passionate about is a form of self-care, which is all about loving and celebrating ourselves.

Some Americans ridicule the concept of self-love. To me, these people are confusing the concept with narcissism. Psychologist Erich Fromm coined the modern use of the term "self-love" in 1956 in his seminal book *The Art of Loving*. To Fromm, loving oneself couldn't be more different from being arrogant, conceited, or egocentric. Loving oneself, he says, involves four acts: caring about oneself, taking responsibility for oneself, respecting oneself, and knowing oneself. The latter, knowing oneself, means being realistic and honest about strengths and weaknesses. How many narcissists do you know who acknowledge their weaknesses, let alone are realistic about them?

To me, loving yourself is not self-indulgent. Taken to extremes, or undertaken mindlessly, I suppose loving yourself could lead to

IDENTIFY AND FOCUS ON IMMEDIATE BENEFITS

My interviewee, fitness trainer Tracy, reminds us that what motivates people to stick with exercise is focusing on the immediate vs. long-term benefits. What are immediate benefits? One is the quality time you get when you work out with a buddy or group. The sense of community is undeniable amongst regular attendees of group exercise classes, whether yoga, zumba, Tai Chi, or boot camp. Other immediate benefits include increased energy, stress reduction, even better sexual performance and stamina. Who doesn't want to have a better time in the sack?

So what's important to you? More energy, less stress, increased productivity, more engagement? Improved happiness? Focus on what motivates you in the short-term, and you're more likely to keep moving your body.

self- indulgence. But many of the people I see in my work as a psychologist and life coach underestimate their value. Doing so leads them into all sorts of trouble, such as entering unsatisfying relationships or taking jobs that deplete them. My definition of self-love includes recognizing that we are of value. We tend to take good care of what is important to us. Our children, our homes, our cars—we take extra good care of these, because they are important to us. Why not extend equal care toward ourselves by exercising more rigorously and eating more healthfully.

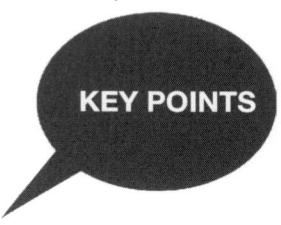

KEY POINTS

- To a person, all those I interviewed agree that self-care is essential to their happiness
- Eating well and getting enough rest and activity provide a foundation in which happiness becomes possible
- Lack of physical activity, poor nutrition, and too much stress and recreational chemicals cause inflammation, which leads to fatigue, grogginess, moodiness, and even anxiety and depression
- Exercise often promotes immediate feelings of euphoria
- A great, natural stress reliever, moving the body can clear the mind and be meditative
- Walking is a great way to boost mood
- How we treat our body and mind today results in how we feel and what we can do tomorrow

PUTTING IT INTO PRACTICE

EXERCISE:

IDENTIFY THE BENEFITS:

Write down the immediate benefits of exercise to you. What does it do for you right away (enjoyment of the outdoors? Seeing a friend? More energy? Increased sex drive?) How do you feel better immediately?

_____

_____

_____

_____

Post these on your bathroom mirror, car dashboard, phone or computer background, or another prominent place.

BEGINNING TO EXERCISE/SIMPLE EXERCISE IDEAS:

Start by walking an additional 10 minutes a day, five out of seven days, for one week. The next week, add an additional 10 minutes a day.
Take the stairs instead of the elevator or escalator.
Park your car at the far end of the parking lot.

FOOD:

SIMPLE SMART FOOD TIPS

ADD MORE OMEGA-3S to your diet. Add in some seafood, eat a handful of nuts a day, sprinkle some seeds like hemp, chia, or flax on salad or cereal. Use olive oil instead of other cooking oils. Take a high-quality fish oil (or other Omega-3) supplement.

Some people complain of a fishy aftertaste to fish oil. Keep the capsules in the freezer, or take them later at night. Vegan options are available; check your nearest health food store.

SUBSTITUTE WHOLE GRAINS for white, bleached, or processed ones. Look for the words "whole grain" on food labels. If it's too much to switch cold turkey, start by mixing them with your current flours.

BLOOD SUGAR STABILIZERS: Increase your consumption of whole grains, root vegetables, and beans and legumes.

Reduce refined sugar, caffeine, and simple carbohydrates (white bread, white rice, white potatoes). Replace these with whole grains, brown rice, and sweet potatoes. If it's too hard to switch at once, start by combining. Perhaps the top slice of bread on that sandwich is your old-time favorite white bread. Place a 100% whole grain one on the bottom. Your taste buds will likely adapt after a week or two, and you can begin experimenting with both slices being whole grain. The friendly counter folks at Chipotle will be glad to give you half white and half brown rice on your burrito or tacos.

WEAN YOURSELF OFF SWEETENERS Replace refined sugar with natural sweeteners, such as local honey or maple syrup, agave nectar, or stevia. Slowly reduce even these. For example, the first week, use one-quarter less honey in your tea. After your taste buds have adjusted, in a week or 10 days, cut that amount by about a quarter. Continue until you can tolerate the taste. That's how I grew to like Green Tea. I couldn't stand the stuff when I first tried it. So I added honey, gradually reducing the amount over time. I now drink one or two cups a day, unsweetened, every day. Avoid artificial sweeteners, as they have been found to negatively impact blood sugar levels.

MEAT REDUCTION Eat meat with most meals? Begin with just replacing one meal a week with a vegetarian entree. Make sure it's something that tastes good to you. Lots of my carnivore friends love meat-free lentil soup. And many folks don't miss the meat in vegetarian Mexican food. All it takes is an open mind, a bit of effort, and some patience.

THE FOOD DIARY Record everything you eat: what, when, how much, and how you feel afterward. After about a week, write the answer to the question, "What am I going to give up and what am I going to substitute?" (this is inspired by President Bill Clinton).

START SMALL Adding even five or ten minutes of walking a day, for example, can make a huge impact on your mood and health.

MAKE JUST ONE SMALL CHANGE AT A TIME Far too many people attempt to make too many changes too fast. Take it slow and easy. You're far more likely to add more healthy habits once one has been established. For instance, when I first started running, after a few good workouts I was naturally motivated to start eating better. When I first starting doing pushups, I congratulated myself for completing ten. Had I aimed for 100 right off the bat, I would have been far more likely to become discouraged and give up.

REWARD YOURSELF Not with a cookie, but in your mind. Tell yourself what a good job you did. Consider success to be making the effort, not seeing the outcome.

TRY FRUIT FOR DESSERT When I first experimented with avoiding processed sugars, I was amazed how quickly my taste buds adapted. Pretty soon, pears seemed sweeter, apples crispier. Even vegetables suddenly revealed their true sweetness. In time, even replacing one dessert a week with fresh fruit can dramatically reduce your caloric intake.

EAT LIKE THE FRENCH I spent Christmas in Paris one year. French cuisine is legendary for good reason; I don't think I ever ate so well. But what most struck me was seeing how the French eat. What they consume may not be considered healthy here (fatty cheeses, white bread baguettes—crunchy outside, soft and chewy inside—with the most delectable strawberry marmalade). But the portions are smaller, and people take their time, really tasting and enjoying the food. Try eating with your full attention, avoiding distractions such as watching TV while you eat. Put your fork down between each bite.

AVOID STRESS

When you're less than perfect, avoid getting down on yourself. In my book (pardon the pun) the stress and emotional damage of self put-downs is worse than the bad habits themselves.

SLEEP For one week, go to bed at the same time and wake up at the same time every day. If you have trouble falling asleep, listen to soothing music or relaxation apps (there are some at my website, www.fullheartliving.com). But stay in bed, even if you're just resting.

Get into the habit of allowing enough time for relaxation and sleep. Put sleep time in your calendar, as you would your work hours. Show up on time, just as you would for work. Stay there until it's time to punch out. (Important note: an exception to this is if you're laying there worrying about falling asleep, which obviously can be counterproductive. I'm talking allowing yourself time to just veg, peacefully. If that's impossible for you, of course get up and do something that might help you relax, such as restorative and certain other forms of yoga.)

Keep a notebook by your bedside. If thoughts occur to you that you don't want to lose, jot them down and then return your mind to relaxation. That way you can let go of trying to remember something.

PUT DOWN YOUR GADGET At least a half hour before bedtime, stop using electronics. Electronic gadgets emit blue light that prevents the release of the hormone melatonin, which is essential for falling and staying asleep.

KEEP A SLEEP DIARY The National Sleep Foundation offers a terrific, free sleep diary that may help shed light on your nocturnal patterns. Visit http://sleepfoundation.org/sleep-diary/SleepDiaryv6.pdf

*This definition was first introduced as a working definition in the World Health Organization paper on 'self-care in the context of primary healthcare' of 2009, and is often referred to as the 'WHO 2009' definition. Webber D, Guo Z, Mann S. Self-care in health: we can define it, but should we also measure it? *SelfCare* 2013;4(5):101-106

**Physical Activity and the Prevention of Depression: A Systematic Review of Prospective Studies, George Mammen, MSc, Guy Faulkner, PhD, *American Journal of Preventive Medicine*, Volume 45, Issue 5, November 2013, Pages 649–657

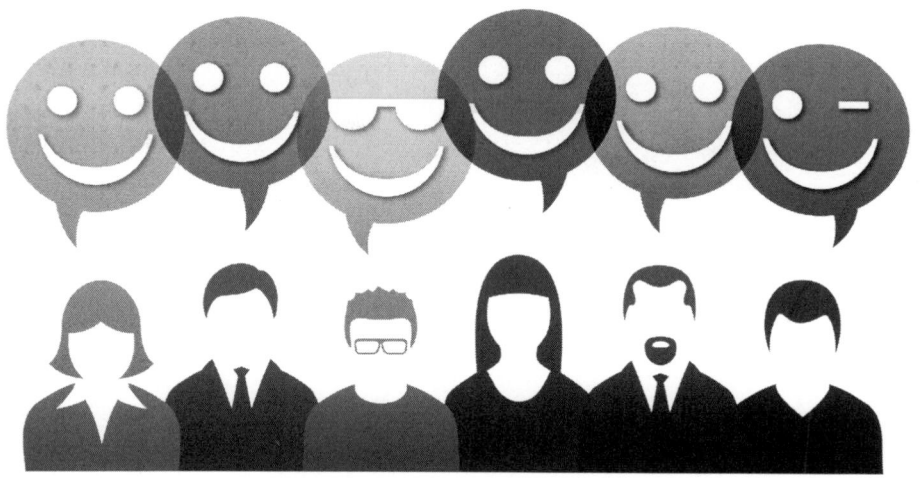

PART TWO

A Happiness
Boot Camp

CHAPTER 5

Expressing thanks:
A poorly wrapped gift

"Key words around happiness are appreciation and gratitude."
  ~ Mia

So here I am, attending to my self-care as faithfully as I can. I am learning how important it is to pay close attention to my sleep, relaxation, food, and exercise. Good, regular sleep is becoming a high priority, and I make time to increase my daily meditation. While allowing myself treats every now and then, I follow Dr. Emmons' nutritional advice carefully. Some form of physical activity makes my to-do list every day. In addition to increasing my happiness, I am beginning to realize that doing these four good things should also increase my life expectancy.

It's true that happiness does make us live longer. At least that is what my colleague, who is an expert in what she calls "Successful Aging," says. I was so impressed with her insights that I book her to be a guest on my live radio show. Two weeks before she is to go on the show, I send her a reminder email.

She replies almost immediately. I am punched breathless when I see the first line. "I am concerned that we have a time conflict." Although my heart is skipping a beat, I continue reading. "Since we set up this date a few months ago, I applied, and was selected, to be a teaching fellow. The teaching fellowship comes with pre-selected dates for meetings. The next meeting is Nov. 22 from 9 a.m. to noon." You guessed it, our show is scheduled for November 22 at 9 a.m., and my colleague can't get out of her meeting.

My chin drops in disbelief. Clearly, she is not all that concerned about this "conflict," as if stating it was all she needed to do. It seems like she's known about being double booked for some time. What if I hadn't emailed her a reminder? What am I supposed to do now! How can I fill a full hour of radio time without a guest?

Trying to take the high road, with just 14 days until the scheduled show date, I send out a flurry of emails to fellow co-hosts to see if they could trade their radio show's time slot for mine. I try to remain calm and hopeful. When it becomes clear no one can trade my time slot, my calm morphs into panic, and I notice I am craving sugar, and I start snapping at my husband and child.

The day of the show is now just seven days away. I sit at my computer with a sinking feeling deep in my gut as I realize that I'm stuck with the original date. My serenity falls. Talk about successful aging—I feel myself aging as I sit here! An internal list of woes begins ("What am I going to do? I don't have a topic or a guest! How could she do this to me?"). I'm shocked to realize I've been breathing shallowly for the past half hour, and my thoughts have become darker and darker. In fact, preoccupied with fear and resentment, I've barely been thinking of my body at all, let alone my breath. So much for good intentions! I close my computer and start to meditate. Relaxing, I breathe in more fully from the diaphragm, allowing my lungs to expand. On the out breath, I release more tension. Slowly in, and slowly out, over and over. It takes my body a full five minutes to return to some semblance of balance.

As my mind begins to clear, an image of my friend Gretchen, the yoga instructor and singer, pops into my mind. She is sitting on a piano bench, wearing a flowing orange top and sporting a nose ring. In her clear, confident voice, I can hear Gretchen saying, "I'm really grateful. And that makes me feel very happy." Her unwavering gaze rivets my attention. "To be really grateful, I think that's what it means to be happy."

GRATITUDE VERSUS APPRECIATION

"Key words around happiness are appreciation and gratitude," Mia says in her videotaped interview. While the two terms often are used interchangeably, gratitude is defined as the quality of being thankful. Taking it a step further, appreciation means recognizing and enjoying the good qualities of someone or something, fully understanding a situation.

Sitting serenely on the couch, smiling, Mia goes further, "Not only just knowing that, but actually letting myself feel it." As she looks down for a second to gather her thoughts, I notice the spring sunshine angling in through the window. Falling on her, the light creates a rainbow aura around her. Mia proceeds, "One of my very excellent yoga teachers says, 'actually feel the sense of contentment.'" So not only think it, but take it a step further by noticing where gratitude and appreciation register inside: "Feel it in your body," Mia implores.

With that message in my head, I get an idea. The show falls on the Saturday before Thanksgiving; why not do a show on gratitude? I pull out the transcripts of my happiness interviews to see if gratitude is a theme in any of them. I realize that gratitude is a thread in nearly all of them. Goodbye successful aging.

Being appreciative of our constant companion, our breath, can actually build happiness. "I feel grateful when I take time to breathe," Gretchen goes on to say. "When I take some time and start there, and recognize that I am alive, and have that gratitude for something so small that in my opinion everything comes out of. It comes out of the breath."

GRATITUDE FOR THE SMILE FROM THE STRANGER ON THE STREET

One day it occurred to fitness trainer Tracy that he wasn't acting out of gratitude. "So I made a decision. I bought this little journal," Tracy tells me. "I carry it with me all the time, and every day I write down something that I'm thankful for. It's a good exercise to write these down."

I wonder how easy this is for him. "Even on bad days?" I ask.

Tracy admits some days are harder; sometimes he has to dig. "Especially on those days, there's still something to be grateful for." At times it can be as simple as being grateful for the smile from the stranger walking down the street, he says.

I can relate. While on my daily run, so often people going the opposite direction make no eye contact. Some of them look wretched, of course, as though every step is painful. I can't blame those people. Struggling, they can barely catch their breath, let alone acknowledge me. But that's rare. Others, with no apparent effort, just seem unfriendly.

The upside is that the un-neighborly ones make it even more noticeable—and pleasurable—when passing runners give me a small wave or, better yet, a hearty, "Good morning!" It just brightens the way a little, providing an extra energy boost. I appreciate friendly runners.

Gretchen feels that awareness of the breath creates a sense of presence. "When I'm breathing, and when I'm able to do that," she says, "it gives me gratitude. And then I look at everything else in a light that is connected, and it makes me feel present. When I'm connected to my breath. And those are the types of things that lead me to continue to grow and be creative."

Having studied with meditation masters and spiritual gurus around the world, Gretchen learned how being grateful for the present moment leads to acceptance. "I'm fortunate that I have the knowledge that the present moment is a manifestation of everything that came before it. So, if I'm grateful for even one thing in this present moment, I have to be self-accepting of everything that happened prior to me being in that moment. So self-acceptance to me is also directly connected to finding gratitude. If you can do that, in the present moment, then you see that everything has led you up to now. To be grateful means to be self-accepting."

Gretchen is referring to an ancient Buddhist teaching, relatively new to many Westerners, often called "Radical Acceptance." Author and meditation teacher Tara Brach defines Radical Acceptance as "the willingness to experience ourselves and our life as it is." Brach endorses Radical Acceptance as "a wholehearted path to freedom."

A SPONTANEOUS MOMENT OF APPRECIATION

Surrounded on three sides by our garden, I was typing on my laptop last June on our screened-in back porch. The beautiful spring sky was clear, and the air was fresh without a trace of humidity. Sounds of occasional planes overhead and road construction less than a block away melted to the background as a gentle breeze flirted with my skin, bringing soothing peace. Breathing it all in, I was grateful for such a perfect moment. What a blessing to be outdoors, writing about happiness—especially in Minnesota, where we are indoors six months out of the year.

As I recall Gretchen's words, I wonder how this might apply to my radio situation. I'm not feeling very accepting of my canceled guest. Nor am I particularly self-accepting of my irritation toward her. How can I be grateful for being placed in such a difficult position, I wonder.

With six days until the radio show, I'm having a hard time holding on to my happiness. I'm making a lot of typos on the computer—and swearing to myself when I do. I'm now really losing my patience with my family. Even the dog is more annoying. Two days in a row I miss my freeway exit. (Yes, the same one!) Irresistible chocolate-mint ice cream cravings randomly erupt. At night, I can barely fall asleep. When at last I do succumb, bad dreams jerk me awake, setting off another round of fretting. True, I now have a good and timely topic, but without an expert guest, I'm worried I can't carry the show on my own. What if I don't do the subject justice? What if I embarrass myself live on air? What if listeners tune out, the station owner yells at me, my co-producers excommunicate me? It doesn't escape me that such ruminations, along with their attendant feelings of resentment—which lead to blaming others—mean I'm living the antithesis of gratitude.

At five days until the show, I have only a rough outline of what I'm going to say. I am beside myself with anxiety. At 2 a.m., unable to sleep, I begin rereading Robert Emmons excellent book *Thanks! How the New Science of Gratitude Can Make You Happier* for ideas on what to talk about. I realize it will take me several days to get enough material to feel comfortable talking about this for a whole hour on the air. Plus the prospect of doing all this work alone overwhelms me. I put *Thanks!* down, and soon fall into a fitful sleep.

THE GRATITUDE JOURNAL

For a month, three times a week, write down one to five things for which you are grateful. Occasionally, include something you tend to take for granted and how you will address that. A simple example might be to offer a silent thanks to the coffee grower whose efforts allowed you to start your morning with that indispensable cup of java. Or you might give appreciation to your partner who takes care of all the yard work. Who knows, you might even be motivated to make or buy him a little gift for his trouble.

The next morning, I wake feeling a little better. I glance at the calendar app on my smartphone. I had been holding time to attend a Friday morning workshop sponsored by a local psychology group, but I knew the group's last meeting had been canceled. Wanting to confirm that this one hasn't also been canned, I surf to the group's website. It turns out the upcoming training was canceled. Damn! Couldn't they have notified me by email weeks ago? Now I've got another thing to be mad at! Nothing's going my way. I thought the deep breaths helped me reduce my irritation, but obviously it's still there, just beneath the surface.

Then I notice the workshop's topic was supposed to have been—get this—"Cultivating Gratitude," and it was to be facilitated by my friend and colleague Patty. I became close friends with Patty when we both were serving on a professional board and teaching a class together. We hadn't been in touch for a while. As I read the description of her workshop, I see that she had published two books and an article on gratitude. If there is such a thing, she's a gratitude expert.

I shoot Patty an email asking if she's interested in being my radio guest this Saturday to talk about gratitude. The next morning, the following message appears in my inbox:

> hi Tom -
> Wow! Thank you for thinking of me! I would be honored to be on your program! Your timing is quite fun: the gratitude scale that my research partner and I have been working on for close to 4 years is completed and just last week our article on it was accepted for publication in the International Journal of Transpersonal Studies! We're not sure of the publication date, but they are going to print it! (eek!)
> I would love to talk with you a bit before then to get a better sense of what you are looking for on the topic. Wow! This feels like such a gift, Tom!
> Thanks!
> Much love,
> ~ Patty

Three days before going live, Patty and I speak by phone and make a plan for what we'll cover. She is an ideal radio guest! At last, I am breathing normally. My irritability vanishes. No more typos, no more missed exits.

The day of the show finally arrives. When I greet her at the studio, I give Patty a big hug—both because it's been at least a year since we've seen each another and out of relief and appreciation. After reminiscing about our teaching days and the board we'd served on, we review the morning's show plan and head in to the sound booth.

"We get so busy and caught up," Patty begins, the show's On-Air light happily beaming at us. "We're almost trained to look at what we don't have. We forget to take a look around at what we actually do have right now. We get lost in all this stuff." As she looks around the studio, she seizes upon the opportunity to provide a concrete, immediate example with what's right in front of her. "Here's this beautiful cup, with hot tea in it."

I ask her to tell us more. Patty says it's important to appreciate even the most everyday things that, in our world of plenty, we often take for granted. She tells the audience that wherever she is, she actively notices and appreciates the good that is near her.

Patty explains that a scarcity mindset, in which we believe we're not good enough or don't have enough, restricts our perspective and leads to suffering. "Gratitude is a shift in perception, when suddenly we're looking at the world as one of abundance. And everything changes. We come alive." I love that last sentence. Gratitude helps us feel alive in a new, vital way.

"Gratitude is an amazing emotion, actually. It's something that you would call a compound, because when we feel gratitude, we tend to feel a lot of other emotions, also," Patty explains. "Joy, love, and hope. When we feel gratitude, it opens us up to this whole realm of positive emotional experiences."

"How do we foster gratitude?" I inquire.

"The interesting thing about gratitude is that it is something we can develop," Patty replies. Listeners wouldn't know it, of course, but I see

Patty's face come alive as she expounds. "We can cultivate it. We can increase it, which then makes it like a skill. So it's a skill, an attitude, and an emotion. It's got it's own unique place, I think, in the realm of human experience."

GRATITUDE FOR WATER

My spiritual teacher, the Venerable Dhyani Ywahoo, who transmits Native American and Buddhist wisdom through Sunray Meditation Society, comes to mind. I first met her at a weekend Peacekeeper workshop held at a YMCA camp deep in the central Minnesota woods. "Water is a sacred element," she says, an essential elixir without which life can't exist. "Give thanks each time you sip water," she instructs, in her lilting, mesmerizing voice, her head tilting toward the nearby lake, just visible through the many oaks and maples that inhabit the camp's land.

"Gratitude is not just a passive feeling," I add, both to clarify and to make sure I understand.

Patty's head nods slightly, and she leans in. "You're right," she affirms. "The deeper we get in to gratitude, the more it becomes a very deeply embodied experience. It can overtake us. When people are feeling gratitude and expressing it, it actually releases oxytocin in the brain." Oxytocin, of course, is the "happy, feel-good" chemical unleashed when we're in love and when parents are holding and bonding with newborn babies. "It's what we crave and desire . . . it's the love transmitter." Wow! I think. Here's a chocolate-free way of obtaining that natural high without the risk of a hefty calorie intake or nasty break-up.

"Gratitude is the antidote to feeling bad," Patty continues. "You can't hold them both very well, because when we're in gratitude we're open to receiving and feeling love." Internally, I list the elements I'm hearing. Gratitude is low-risk, doesn't cost anything, transmits love, and helps counter feeling bad. Seems like a win-win to me.

I ask if there is anything else about gratitude that surprised her or stands out. "Yes, another thing about gratitude that's really unique," Patty says in the show, "is, it's really, by definition, a relational experience. We experience it in response to something or someone." So there's an interactive component to it. We're not simply passive recipients; we're engaged and involved.

THE APPRECIATION LETTER

To deepen your expression of gratitude, consider writing a thank you letter to your favorite teacher, mentor, chef, newscaster, doctor, bus driver, author, or librarian. Be specific. Tell them what they did and how what they did impacted you—and how they continue to influence you today. This isn't a place for criticisms of any kind. Only include positives. To take it a step further, deliver your letter in person, and read it aloud. Notice how you feel and how the person responds.

Although we need others to cultivate gratitude, "we seem to be very skilled at blaming our relationships," Patty says. "I wouldn't have to be unhappy if he would just do this or that"—we can so easily believe—"or if my boss did this, or if I had a better job. I would feel better if I were taller, thinner, then my life would be full of whatever, this abundance."

"I have a great example of blame for you, Patty," I say. "At the beginning of every season, my husband and I argue over the thermostat. No matter what, it seems I'm too hot, he's too cold, or vice versa. Life would be so much easier if he just adhered to my temperature needs!"

"That's a great example of focusing on blame and not abundance," Patty concurs. "Because how wonderful it is that we have the ability to regulate the temperature in our houses. That's almost like magic. We go outside, we can't control the temperature. Inside, there's a little box that you can push or turn and suddenly—it's cool. That's abundance!"

My spine tingles as I put the pieces together. When I focus only on my preferences, and me, I can get stuck in resentment. If I look more broadly, I can be grateful for the thermostat, the furnace, my home and my husband. The list of things to be grateful for may be infinite. When I invite myself to honor the positives, I feel better. Greg and I may still need to negotiate the air conditioning settings from time to time. Coming from gratitude, however, I'm much more likely to state my needs in a way Greg can hear, increasing the chance that we'll arrive at a compromise that works and sustain our relationship.

SAYING GRACE

One mild, overcast winter day, my friend Trena and I meet for lunch at the Lowry, one of my favorite Minneapolis haunts. As the server gently sets our sandwiches and salads in front of us, Trena suddenly asks, "Do you say grace before eating?"

"Not formally," I reply. "When I remember, I tend to give thanks silently."

Trena nods and then bows her head as she gives thanks in her way. I, too, pause for a moment, considering all that went in to this plate of sustenance before me: From the miracle of photosynthesis to the farmer, the truck driver, the grocer, the chef, the server, and more, a series of events—all of which require effort—took place so that I can receive nourishment. Trena and I continue our meal and conversation. As we do, however, I notice a shift. Though our prayer was unspoken, sharing a moment of silence before digging in made each bite and each word following more precious.

After the radio show is over, it occurs to me that I could try applying these concepts to my originally scheduled guest. True, her eleventh-hour cancelation annoyed and inconvenienced me, and my scrambling to find a replacement resulted in anxiety. However, it's pretty incredible that I have a radio show at all. As Patty would say, "That's abundance!" That's when it came to me. My original guest's cancelation turned into "a poorly wrapped gift." What looks unappealing on the outside can sometimes be the most valuable once it's fully unwrapped.

The next time something like this happens, hopefully I can remember what I learned from this experience, curb my reactivity, and look for gifts. I see now that I could have viewed the challenge as an opportunity instead of a hassle. Doing so, I suspect, would have helped me trust that even if Patty hadn't miraculously come through for me, I would have figured something out without making my family miserable or resorting to junk food.

Perhaps that's what Radical Acceptance means. The incredible experience of exploring gratitude on the show made me realize how thankful I am to my originally scheduled guest. If she hadn't dropped out, I wouldn't have had these epiphanies or had the chance to reconnect with Patty. And I might not have had the pleasure and good fortune of learning about gratitude from a true expert.

KEY POINTS

KEY POINTS

- Gratitude is a skill that can be cultivated
- Being grateful releases oxytocin, the "feel good," relational chemical
- Expressing thanks can provide a potent antidote to feeling bad
- Being grateful can lead to Radical Acceptance, the willingness to experience ourselves and our life as they are
- When feeling thankful, we are open to receiving love
- Experienced in response to something or someone, gratitude by definition, is a relational experience
- Gratitude can contribute to growth and creativity

PUTTING IT INTO PRACTICE

ADVANCED APPRECIATION PRACTICE

See if you can write two to three sentences about an experience of gratitude. The aim is increased awareness of what you appreciate, why, how it registers inside, and how you are an active participant.

1. **IDENTIFY** Notice what you are grateful for.
2. **EXPAND** Notice more deeply. What specifically are the qualities or the elements you appreciate?
3. **EXPLORE** What does this experience tell or teach you? What does it mean to you?
4. **DEEPEN** How do you respond? How do you acknowledge it? How did you take it in?
5. **BRING IT FULL CIRCLE** How are you a participant in this whole experience? What do you contribute?

Use this template to write about your gratitude experience:

1. **IDENTIFY** I am grateful for

_____

_____

_____

_____

_____

_____

2. **EXPAND** The qualities or elements I appreciate about the above include

_____

_____

_____

_____

_____

_____

3. EXPLORE This teaches me and/or brings meaning to me by

_____

_____

_____

_____

_____

_____

4. DEEPEN I respond, acknowledge, and take this in by

_____

_____

_____

_____

_____

_____

5. BRING IT FULL CIRCLE I am an active participant and contribute to this experience by

_____

_____

_____

_____

_____

_____

START THE DAY WITH THANKSGIVING Over your morning coffee or tea, take a moment to consider what you're grateful for and how you help manifest that. Like Patty, we might be grateful for the cup and warm beverage in our hand. Many mornings, my first thought is how thankful I am for the gift of a good night's sleep. You might appreciate the moments of quiet before the day gets in full swing, your friendly neighborhood barista, or the morning newspaper.

BREATH BREAK If you can, take a few moments throughout the day to breathe deeply. In your mind, acknowledge the gifts of the day or the moment. What's going well right now?

SAY GRACE before meals. See if you can take a moment before meals. If not a formal prayer, simply reflect on all the effort that went into bringing this food to you, from the miracle of photosynthesis to the farmers, truck drivers, grocer, and cook who participated in bringing it to your plate. This can be done either silently or aloud—or both!

DRINKING WATER Before taking a sip of water, give a silent word of thanks for it.

BREATHE in gratitude. Imagine it going to every cell. When grateful, imagine you can feel it with your whole body.

SMILE to people you pass, and be grateful for their smiles in return.

VALIDATE OTHERS' THANKS When someone thanks you, look them in the eye. Take a breath. Smile and say, "You're welcome." And mean it.

THE GRATITUDE STROLL Take a walk letting your senses be the guide, and notice all the things for which you are grateful. These might include the fresh air, the shape of the clouds, the evergreens in the park, the fit of your favorite shoes, the aroma from your neighbor's grill, the buzz of insects, or countless other things. (Inspired by Marelisa Fabrega)

FOUR QUESTIONS At or near the end of each day, ask yourself one or all of these:
- What touched me today?
- Who or what inspired me today?
- What made me smile today?
- What's the best thing that happened today?

(Inspired by Marelisa Fabrega)

GRATITUDE MEDITATION Take a few moments to settle in. Close your eyes if you like. Notice how your breath affects your body. Perhaps become aware of the rise and fall of the belly, or the expansion and contraction of the chest, or the movement of air in your nostrils. After a few moments, if it's comfortable, move your awareness to your heart. With each breath, imagine breathing in gratitude, all the way in to your heart. With each out breath, imagine breathing out gratitude, from the very depths of your heart. Allow the gratitude to sink deeply into your heart. Allow gratitude to flow freely from your heart. When you're ready, on an in breath, allow the gratitude to sink deeply into your whole body. And allow gratitude to flow freely from your entire body on the out breath. Remain in this state for as long as you like. End with a dedication such as, "May all beings know freedom from suffering. May all beings be happy. May all beings be free." (Inspired by Thich Nhat Hanh)

CHAPTER 6

Developing mindfulness: Happiness is a state of consciousness

Minnesota, of course, is well known for legendary weather extremes. Proud of our fortitude, we Minnesotans revel in the fact that our summer heat and winter snow keep the population down.

In my early 30s, I lived in a high-rise along Minneapolis' Greenway. This gorgeous outdoor corridor connects downtown with Loring Park, and is aptly named for its many evergreens, towering maples, and other growing things. While I was thrilled that I could walk the 10 or so blocks to work in the Medical Arts Building, late one spring it occurred to me that the season had almost passed and I'd barely noticed that the trees I passed every day were green again. So caught up in my thoughts about the day to come—or on the way home, replaying what had happened that day—that I was oblivious to the beauty right in front of me.

Every one of the happy folks I interview, on the other hand, talks about the opposite of obliviousness, namely, mindfulness. Not all of them call it mindfulness. Some refer to it as "tuning in" or "waking up," some "presence" or "conscious living" or "savoring the moment." But all of them speak of some form of heightened awareness of the present moment.

As a hairdresser and salon owner, Warren interacts with perhaps hundreds of people a week. "I don't see a lot of people walking around with a general sense of self-awareness," he says. "You know, they're sort of just skirting through life, just making it. I can't think of the word. Mindless, maybe. Just through rote." Like me, blind to spring budding all around me.

With all due apologies to the many phenomenal teachers out there, I always compare mindlessness with being in school. Who hasn't sat through a boring lecture and found themselves thinking of something else. Maybe you replay a scene from the latest Batman movie in your mind, or you draft your grocery list. Driving down the freeway, you might go on autopilot, so deep in thought you miss your exit. These are examples of "tuning out."

As Warren explains during his interview, in his deep, resonant voice, "They are not present in their moment. Their mind is somewhere else. They are not focused on what is going on in that moment."

With mindfulness, conversely, you're fully absorbed in an activity; the mind is distraction-free. Happy people do this a lot.

In his interview, wearing his signature brown hoodie and sporting a few days' beard, Detroiter Philip particularly captures my attention when he says, "The degree with which we are engaged directly contributes to the happiness we have in our lives. How tuned are you to your surroundings? Ultimately that steers my personal happiness, the level of engagement. It's very easy to become unaware, because there's Facebook, petty things. Maybe there's somebody driving slow in front of you, so you miss some things.

"Being tuned in means being fully aware of your surroundings," Philip continues. "It's almost an impossible thing to be at 100 percent. But as we increase our level of engagement with the things around us, suddenly we become happier."

High Touch over High Tech

Listen to this 20-something, who grew up with home computers and cellular telephones, on technology: "When you're able to walk to work and able to just listen to the things around you, not listen to your iPod," Philip says, "that is directly correlated to happiness. When you have a moment to yourself, within the surroundings that exist, that's when we get to happiness."

Minneapolis therapist Mia, sitting comfortably on the couch in her pearls and flowing white top, says it well during her interview. "When I am fully in the here and now, I'm not thinking about 'Oh, I shouldn't have said that yesterday,' or 'What am I going to say tomorrow?' Instead, I'm like, 'Oh, I'm here with you saying this,' and letting that be okay."

THE WORLD AT YOUR FEET

"You need not leave your room. Remain sitting at your table and listen. You need not even listen, simply wait. You need not even wait, just learn to become quiet, and still, and solitary. The world will freely offer itself to you to be unmasked. It has no choice; it will roll in ecstasy at your feet."
~Franz Kafka

Mia asserts that this state of mind is essential to her happiness. "When I am fully in the here and now, happiness is available." I suspect that Mia is saying she appreciates the fullness of the here and now. Not wanting to be somewhere else, not dreaming of what might be, not wishing things had been different in the past. She's in the present moment, right now—100 percent.

During filming, Gretchen, folding her long legs in front of her, agrees. Heightened awareness is not only necessary for this singer and yoga instructor's happiness, it's how she defines it. To her, happiness means, "whether I'm feeling elated and laughing and smiling, or I'm feeling some sense of sorrow for something and crying—I allow myself to feel those emotions and just be present. Through that honesty and truthfulness, that's where happiness is. It's not all about laughter."

That sentiment is part of what prompted me to ask about the juxtaposition of happiness and sadness. So many people seem unclear on this.

In a moment of adolescent angst, I remember writing this note to my 16-year-old self: "I am searching for a constant state of happiness."

"Grief Is Cleansing"

Thirty-plus years later, "It's okay to be down or sad at times?" I ask Dr. Emmons.

"I think it's not only okay. I think it can be really cleansing." He offers grief as an example. "It is an emotion that we are simply meant to have. If we can really feel our sadness, and our grief and our loss, then it's as if it simply washes over us and through us."

He looks away for a moment. "It can leave us feeling in some way cleansed, and in some way strengthened. So absolutely welcoming the whole range of emotions, I think, is really important." What a great way to think of our emotional lives. Sadness and grief are cleansing. We rinse berries before we eat them to rid them of any impurities. Our feelings, likewise, help us rinse our souls of impurities.

The same thing is true, Dr. Emmons says, with thoughts—which link to our feelings.

"If you become more aware of what is going on in your mind at any given moment, you'll begin to see the connection between your thoughts and your emotions. If you pay close attention when you're feeling bad, it's usually associated with something you were thinking."

I can come up with countless examples of this in my own life. Just the other day I was scrubbing away at the kitchen sink. Now, friends often tease me about my cleanliness habits. I wouldn't say I'm obsessive-compulsive, but I like things clean. So I was working hard. (Okay, maybe I do have some OCD tendencies when it comes to cleaning.)

Unbidden, one of my most "stuck" former clients came to mind. This suffering soul thought he could be happy only if everything he did was accomplished perfectly. Whenever I tried to point out what was good about him—despite his having done something that didn't meet his high expectations—he resisted. No matter what I said, he remained convinced that he was not lovable or acceptable. I suspect my perfectionistic dish washing reminded me of him. I could feel myself starting to feel guilty that I had been unable to help him much.

Dr. Emmons' ideas shed light. "Being able to really monitor our thoughts," he explains, "doesn't stop us from having negative or bad thoughts—at least I think you have to be very advanced to be able to do that—but it does allow you to respond to those thoughts consciously, by choice. You can choose whether you act on them, believe them, entertain them, or keep having them over and over again, if you're conscious of them. And that makes a very big difference about how we feel."

Applying that wisdom, as I was drying my hands, I was able to reassure myself. Yes, that particular client didn't improve much. But that doesn't mean I'm a bad psychologist. I don't have to catch his "self-hatred fever." Awareness of my thoughts and emotions helped me get back to more important matters, like appreciating the view from my kitchen window. Or disinfecting doorknobs.

Cultivating Mindfulness

So where does mindfulness come from? How do we develop it?

Being free of recreational chemicals is an important component for artist Jenn. "It's not that I was addicted," she explains. "It's that I was abusive. I would drink once a week but I couldn't have one. I had to have a bunch. And I'd be hung over the next day, and the next two days I would be depressed. So that's four, three-and-a-half days out of my life that I wasn't as present as I possibly could be. And that right now is the most important thing." She looks determined and hopeful.

Travel helps Philip. "Travel puts me in this unfamiliar setting that's completely unknown, and I start observing very closely the things around me. Paying attention to all these little things, I get into this state of mind where I become sensitized again. So suddenly the things that create my daily existence here are looked at in a very different light."

I, too, find I appreciate home more after having been away even for just a few days. The dog seems fluffier, my pillow comfier, the grass a deeper shade of green.

Dr. Emmons says mindfulness can be found anywhere. He has a caveat, however. "I think that it is very, very helpful to have some kind of a formal practice of mindfulness or awareness in the form of meditation.

"It doesn't have to just be one type of meditation," Dr. Emmons continues. Having sampled dozens of forms of meditation, including singing, chakra awareness, Qi Gong, and hours of silent sitting, this grabs my attention.

"I think what's called Mindfulness Meditation is a really, really good way to do it," Dr. Emmons continues, his voice exuding calm and reassurance—which tells me he practices what he preaches. "But you could bring mindful awareness into walking. Walking meditation is a good way to go about this for people who have trouble sitting for a long period of time or who get distracted. It's nice to have something physical. You can even do it through other forms of movement like Tai Chi or yoga, because if you're doing it consciously, that can become a meditative practice, building your skill of awareness.

"Do it over and over again," he instructs, "because things will occur that will take you out of awareness, and you just have to keep bringing yourself back." I know all about that. I used to wonder if I could ever call myself a meditator given how unwieldy my mind can be when I try to slow it down.

"Meditation is just a very useful short cut, if you will, to being able to develop greater awareness," Dr. Emmons continues. "Because as you sit, you'll have numerous opportunities to bring yourself back. As we begin a practice like this, the mind is really, really good at distracting us, at taking us somewhere else. In my view, that's not really a problem. The key is to just notice that you've done that and keep bringing yourself back. That's the practice of mindfulness, and that's where you really strengthen that ability."

So cultivating mindfulness can come from travel. Closer to home, meditation, whether sitting or movement-based, can help. You can even take a class.

Appalled to realize that I was missing Minnesota's glorious seasons, almost 20 years ago I took an eight-week course in mindfulness. Based on the Mindfulness Based Stress Reduction program developed by Jon Kabat-Zinn, we learned silent meditation, body scans, and yoga. We breathed. We practiced being fully in the present moment.

Since then, whether walking to work or glancing out the window, when the trees change, I notice.

KEY POINTS

KEY POINTS

- Mindfulness is full attention in the present moment, free of distractions and judgments
- While they might call it different things, everyone I interviewed practices mindfulness
- Mindfulness can help you connect to yourself and to others
- Mindfulness can help with problem solving
- Any activity can be performed mindfully
- Especially when first learning mindfulness, many people prefer movement vs. stationary meditations

PUTTING IT INTO PRACTICE

LET GO of seeking a constant state of happiness. Embrace the fullness of every moment, even the less desirable ones. When you're sad, for instance, be sad. Like all emotions and experiences, it will come and go. While it often seems counterintuitive, the more you resist, the longer the unwanted feeling or experience is likely to last. Support yourself to tolerate whatever is occurring right now.

START BY JUST NOTICING Most of us "tune out" occasionally as a means of coping with the demands of modern life. Notice when you're tuning out, and make it a conscious choice instead of something done automatically without your permission. Do you truly need some down time right now? Have your down time with your full awareness. Conversely, might you be missing something really important just now? I'll never forget hearing about a mother who kept asking her young daughter to hurry up so they could get to school or other important places. When it came time for her daughter to leave home at age 18, in her need to get places on time, the mother realized she'd missed too many precious moments. Only when her daughter was grown did she realize that punctuality is not as important as her daughter.

IDENTIFY PATTERNS AND THEMES Keep a log of when you tend to tune out. What are you doing? Watching TV? Driving? What does that tell you?

GO FOR A WALK As you walk, notice how your foot feels as it strikes and leaves the ground. What sights, sounds, and aromas come to you? Your mind will inevitably be drawn to other matters, such as your to-do list or a recent argument. When that happens, just notice it, and return your attention over and over again to your five senses. In this way, simply walking—with full attention—becomes a meditation.

FOCUS ON WHAT'S HAPPENING RIGHT NOW When your mind wanders, simply return your focus to what is right in front of you. You're likely to have to do this repeatedly. It takes time to train the mind to stay in one place.

For a week, **CHOOSE ONE MUNDANE ACTIVITY**, like brushing your teeth or walking up the stairs. Each time you engage in that action, bring your full attention to it. When your mind wanders, gently steer it back.

BRING YOUR FULL ATTENTION TO ANY PHYSICAL ACTIVITY Many people find sitting meditation difficult, especially at the beginning. Moving the body can help. Experiment with bringing your full attention to any physical activity you're doing, whether swimming, biking, gardening, lifting, or whatever it is you do with your body.

REDUCE THE USE OF ELECTRONICS Useful and compelling as they can be, electronic devices can reinforce the tendency to drift away from the present moment. Use them selectively, and be as mindful as you can while you do so. Think "High Touch" over "High Tech"—how can I be most in touch with myself while I use this equipment?

GET OUTSIDE The act of being in nature is soothing and meditative for most of us, especially if we fully experience being outside, instead of listening to the constant chatter in our minds.

ATTEND TO YOUR LOVED ONES When in the presence of others, especially those most important to you, give them your full, undivided attention. Listen fully and speak sparingly and only from the heart. More of this in Chapter 9: Connecting.

TAKE A MINDFULNESS-BASED STRESS REDUCTION (MBSR) COURSE This is the best way I know for Westerners unfamiliar with meditation to learn all kinds of ways to be more fully in the present moment.

TAKE A MOVEMENT-BASED CLASS High-quality classes such as Tai Chi, Qi Gong, and yoga are phenomenal for teaching moment-by-moment awareness.

READ A skeptic? Read Dan Harris' amazing book *10% Happier: How I Tamed the Voice in My Head, Reduced Stress Without Losing My Edge, and Found Self-Help That Actually Works—A True Story*. After suffering a panic attack on live national television, Harris was desperate for drastic change. Though he'd been suspicious of meditation his whole life, this highly public crisis eventually led him to a deep exploration of mindful meditation. He tells the harrowing yet gripping tale with the wit and grit only a seasoned journalist can muster.

CHAPTER 7

Celebrating simple joys: The passion of sandpapering blankets

Ryan is a clean-cut, 20-something with an adorable smile. With his hectic schedule, it's easiest for him to make his way to my office for his interview one sunny, early spring weekday. As he settles on the couch, I am struck once again by how well put together he appears. As always, his clothing seems well pressed, his face looks freshly shaven, and he appears confident, calm, and well rested.

One of my favorite moments from our time together involves his tale of a short film he made in college. It was a spoof on a once popular fabric softener commercial. In Ryan's film, the main character takes her favorite childhood blanket out of the dryer only to find it anything but soft. In fact, it comes out of the dryer torn and tattered.

There was one problem. He had purchased a brand-new blanket. "I had to make it look old," Ryan says. "So I tacked it onto a cork-board, and I took some sandpaper and I'm just going like this." Ryan's right palm makes quick circles in the air. "As I was doing it, I realized, 'This is how you make movies. It's this right here, doing stuff like this.'"

Many people think filmmaking is glamorous and sexy. But as Ryan well knows, "it's about moments like that, where you got this little blanket, you've got sandpaper and you're trying to rough it up. If you can enjoy those moments, then you're on the right track. And I did, because I saw where it was going."

Passion, then, is key. Ryan knew that shredding that blanket, onerous though the chore may have seemed, was in reality a step on his quest to become a filmmaker. "If you take it out of context, how could you find enjoyment in that?" he asks. I see what he means. How often is ruining a blanket fun? Ryan learned to put such menial tasks into perspective. "I came to understand it's part of something larger," he tells me.

It's hard to believe just two years prior, this busy go-getter could barely drag himself off the couch. Ryan's shoulders drop as he tells me more about that dark time. He says the problem actually started a lot further back. He believes it began when he was labeled "gifted" as a young child. "I always felt this pressure that I was going to do something great." Nothing particularly spectacular happened in high school, however, so surely he would do something remarkable in college.

He entered the University of Minnesota not knowing what he wanted as his major. "The reason I went to the 'U' was that they have every major. When I figure out what I want to do, they're going to have it,'" he recalls thinking.

Without direction, however, Ryan floundered. He spent a lot of time partying. "I failed a couple classes because I just wasn't showing up." This continued for about two years. Like his grades, his self-esteem plummeted.

"It got to the point where my parents, my dad specifically, saw me as a failure. And obviously that was hard to take. I should have reached out to my parents because I needed help." I hear the pain and shame in Ryan's voice.

He realized that every night it was the same torment. "I'd lay down to go to bed and I would think to myself, 'Did I accomplish anything of merit today?' And it was very frustrating when, no, I didn't." Feeling he was without prospects, hope dwindling, Ryan started not sleeping.

He was lost. "I didn't know what the next step was." During this terrible time, he was watching a lot of movies. But he wasn't watching them mindlessly. In fact, he took copious notes while watching films. "And then one day it hit me," Ryan's face brightens as he sits up straighter. "Watching this film, there were people behind that camera. There were people who got paid to make movies. From there, my life was altered."

Ryan enrolled in acting and directing classes. Eventually quitting school, he began making movies. Today, in addition to producing and directing his own films, he is a professional crowd-funding coordinator and runs the Minneapolis 48 Hour Film Project, in which teams compete to see who can make the best short film in only 48 hours.

Discovering that film was his passion cured Ryan's depression and insomnia. Not sleeping is no longer an issue. "Now I'm exhausted," he boasts. "Because I'm so busy, there are so many things going on that at the end of the day, I just crash." A far cry from his days on the couch— and sleepless nights—only a few years prior.

Dr. Emmons weighs in on this idea. "I think paying attention to what really feeds us brings us life. It's a really good way to make ourselves happier. It is a great antidote to stress." And he provides a warning about self-improvement: "A lot of times people get caught up in trying to improve themselves. It's a different way of approaching this than the approach of doing something you really love. Because if you're working on improving yourself, it implies there's something wrong that you need to fix. Whereas if you're really looking at filling your life with things that bring you joy, things that you love, then it's possible to live in such a vibrant way. Focusing on things that really give us life is a really smart thing to do."

I think of people I know who have that joyful focus. I see it in my son when he plays basketball. He loves the sport for many reasons, including the mental and physical challenge, teamwork, satisfaction of playing his best, and roar of the crowd after seamlessly sinking a three-pointer.

But Dr. Emmons says there's more to it. I ask him if he is referring to the state of "flow," defined by Mihaly Csikszentmihalyi in his book *Flow: The Psychology of Optimal Experience* as "a mental state in which a person is fully immersed or engaged in an activity."

"If you're in a state of flow, you don't lose yourself, exactly," Dr. Emmons comments. "I think you lose your small self—the ego, the conscious self. When you're really in a state of flow, those little things that we often think are so important, they just fade. They go by the wayside. We're just in that moment completely."

It may sound overly simple, but Dr. Emmons believes, "If we can really be completely present to whatever is—whether that is something we like or something we don't like—it is in that presence that we really have our power. How we respond to it. We have our choices that we can make." (See Chapter 6: Developing mindfulness, for greater detail on this concept.)

Ryan is in good company among those I interviewed. Each of my interviewees has particular passions and engages in them often. One of Mia's top passions is baking pies. She doesn't make them just for herself, however. She bakes them fresh and brings them to friends. She chooses which of her ceramic pie plates to use based on the recipient's favorite color. Gretchen sings. Dr. Emmons loves to spend hours in his garden. Tracy coaches soccer. Jenn makes sculptures and is a photographer.

As Jenn tells me in her light-filled Minneapolis apartment, "I have my son. I have my life. I have great friends. I have air to breathe and I have birds to listen to. Yeah. It's a great place to be where I am right now. Every day it's challenging, you know. But you just kind of keep going. I know that tomorrow I'll be there, I'll be here." Engaging in her passions helps her appreciate even the seemingly mundane.

"I don't see a separation between work and life," Ryan says. "For me they're one in the same because I enjoy immensely what I'm doing. I feel like I'm always working because I'm always living. It's choosing things you love to do. I don't see a lot of people doing that. Think for yourself. Ask yourself, what do I want, and then go for it, because you only live once. If it's always easy, then the rewards are not nearly as great."

As the poet Rumi said, "Let yourself be silently drawn by the strange pull of what you really love." So what do you really love? What is your strange pull? Are you heeding its silent call?

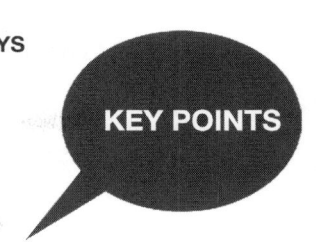
KEY POINTS

KEY POINTS

- Engaging one's passions brings deep pleasure
- Valuing the simplest moments contributes to joy
- Happy people appreciate how such moments are part of a greater plan
- Taking risks supports happiness
- Happier people are true to themselves
- Beware of self-improvement if it only reinforces the belief that something is wrong with you. Instead, approach change from a place of self-love
- Focusing on what brings joy is a potent antidote to difficulties and challenges

PUTTING IT INTO PRACTICE

ENJOY THE SIMPLE MOMENTS How can you make doing the laundry fun? Sing along to the radio, or chat with a friend on the phone while you fold. Hate mowing the lawn? Create different patterns in the grass. This idea (and he has many more) is from my friend and colleague Andy Weisberg's book *Laid Off and Crazy Happy*.

RECALL ON THE GREATER PLAN Making lunch for the kids? Think of how that peanut butter is going to fuel your daughter's brain for learning tomorrow afternoon. Maybe it will provide just the jolt she needs to decide to become the next president!

REDISCOVER YOUR PASSIONS When you were young, how did you answer the question, "What do you want to do be when you grow up?" What activities did you most enjoy? Answering these questions will likely lead you to what would be most enjoyable for you now.

Once you know where your interests lie, **TAKE A CLASS, JOIN A CLUB**, or **VOLUNTEER** in that area.

ALLOW YOURSELF TO TAKE RISKS If the above seems too scary, explore how you could support yourself to follow through. Maybe you need a friend to come along. Perhaps you don't believe you deserve to have fun. If so, refute the irrational part of the belief. Remind yourself you **DO** have the right to enjoy yourself.

BE TRUE TO YOURSELF Are there areas of your life where you are violating your own values? Perhaps you're not as honest as you'd like to be. How can you begin to live with more integrity? Choose one relationship to start. Be more truthful with that person. Notice how you feel.

PUT DOWN THAT SELF HELP BOOK Even this one! If you're trying to change out of self-hatred, you are far more likely to fail. If you start from a place of love and acceptance of yourself, you're far more likely to succeed.

CHAPTER 8

Accepting yourself:
Half off the beaten path

Dr. Emmons likes to cite his favorite lines by 13th century Persian poet, Rumi: "'Half of any person is wrong and weak and off the beaten path. Half! The other half is dancing and swimming and laughing in the invisible joy!'

"It's a great quote," he says, and adds, "It's a way of acknowledging that we've got sides to ourselves that struggle. The suffering is there. We carry it, and we're not always good at doing these things that we're talking about. But there's another side of us that's always able to tap into this joy that is always present. I think it really speaks to the human condition in a very honest way, in a way that summarizes everything we've been talking about in terms of happiness."

I can't help but feel excited. He's right, of course. It is a great quote. While part of life—Rumi says half—is struggle, the other half is joy! It sheds light on one of life's great paradoxes: we are divided creatures. We are ashamed of some parts of ourselves, while we take pride in other parts. This divisive nature often leads to inner conflict, with one side pulling against the other.

One source of shame for me is my tendency to get defensive when I feel I am being judged, regardless of whether the criticism is justified or unjustified. In time, I came to realize that this habit is connected to my history of being bullied at school.

The bullying started in seventh grade when a handful of boys labeled me "gay." As early as five years old, I knew my interests were more aligned with what girls often liked, but I never put a name to it. As I grew older, I had inklings that our culture considered it "bad." By the time I was in junior high school, I was a confused adolescent (what adolescent isn't?!), so when I heard that first slur, I was utterly stunned. How could they call me that? I knew it was "bad," but I wasn't even sure myself if it applied to me. Like stumbling onto a hidden landmine, I was completely unprepared.

While everyone seemed to know I was different, no one had ever told me that this difference might result in being bullied. I didn't know how to respond. All I knew to do was what my dad had taught me whenever there was a problem: ignore it, and hope it goes away. But the hateful name-calling didn't go away. If anything, it got worse. Those ignorant, sneering, pubescent homophobes added more slurs: "faggot, pansy ass, queer, ladies' man." But "fag" was by far their favorite. And even if I didn't at first know each term's precise meaning, there was no doubt their slurs were pejorative, and they all implied that I wasn't man enough.

One of the hardest parts was that I had no warning. From the moment I stepped out of the house, I knew there was potential for humiliation. At any time or place I could be targeted. Whether stepping onto the bus, walking down the hallway, or entering a classroom, one or more of these boys could publicly humiliate me. I felt completely exposed and unsafe, and no adult seemed to care.

Whenever these bully incidents occurred, I wanted to shrink into a crack in the industrial-strength cinder block wall or evaporate into thin air. Often the verbal abuse was accompanied by threats of physical harm. "You better watch out, kid. We're gonna whoop your gay ass." (At the time, it didn't occur to me to wonder why they were so interested in my hind parts.)

I didn't talk to anyone about it; I didn't know how. Back then bullying wasn't recognized for the crippling power it can wield. Desperate, I wracked my brain for what I was doing to cause this relentless torment. I felt the only solution was that I had to change. I tried everything and anything I could think of: I started holding my books at my side ("only girls hold their books at chest level"), not speaking ("don't draw attention to yourself!"), smoking cigarettes ("that'll make me look cool"). Nothing helped. Finally, feeling utterly powerless and mortified, and having no one to talk to about it, the only option was to believe that there must be something wrong with me. Thus the bullying beliefs began to release their soul poison; I began to believe "this is my fault for being who I am. I deserve this." Helplessness became my default *modus operandi*. This is how shame penetrates. As kids, we don't even know it is happening.

Nearly all of us endure some sort of shaming as kids. For many of us, such shaming experiences don't fade with time as many other memories do. Instead, shame memories linger in a special region of the brain where, even into adulthood, they can be triggered. For me, all someone has to do is "sigh" at something I say, and immediately I go on red alert; I believe I must have done something bad or wrong. It doesn't matter if the criticism is warranted or imagined, right or wrong. Either I shut down, withdrawing to protect myself, or I go into attack mode and justify my actions. When this happens, of course, I am not fully being present. Worse, I barely recognize myself.

I am learning what I need to do when I sense a red alert has been triggered. I need to accept my feelings of fear, anger, and powerlessness as simply that: feelings. I don't have to go into emotional flight or fight.

Remaining in the present moment, I can accept that I am off my well-beaten path and wandering into my own private jungle. Accepting that my feelings have derailed me—and not beating myself up for it—provides a safety mechanism. Such acceptance and self-compassion provide the emotional and mental footing needed to get back onto the path where I can make mindful instead of instinctual choices. Even (or perhaps particularly) when I am alarmed, I strive to take in what others are saying and to keep an open mind and an open heart. Only then can I take responsibility for anything I may have done. Once I can accept my part, I can start to see what I need to do. When I am connecting with myself like this, I can connect with others—and nothing makes me happier.

Rumi's quote reveals the essence of the existential question that brings many into therapy: "Do I need to accept myself as I am, or do I need to change?" The paradoxical answer is, of course, both. Only by embracing the truth of what I am doing now can I make lasting change. Accepting what is happening allows the change process to unfold. This is a key point. Long before 12-step groups made it so popular, one of my dad's favorite quotes was Reinhold Niebuhr's Serenity Prayer:

God, grant me the serenity to accept the things I cannot change,
The courage to change the things I can,
And the wisdom to know the difference.

This prayer reminds me that I have no control over other people, and I do not control many of the circumstances I find myself in. I am, however, in full charge of my responses.

It's important to distinguish between our reactions and our responses. Reactions refer to our immediate sensations and feelings. Responses are what we actually do, how we act—our behaviors. Here's an example from my own life. Having experienced bullies' severe and unfair criticism during adolescence, I may later often react (i.e., have sensations and feelings) defensively when I feel criticized or judged. How I respond—what I do with those feelings—is where I can initiate change. I can practice yoga breathing to stay calm, for example, or I might say, "I hear what you're saying, let me get back to you on that."

Accepting the fact that my defensive reaction arises gives me the emotional traction to choose how I respond. I can consciously decide to stay open and not shut down. Rumi's poem provides permission to hold and honor both these parts of myself: the struggling, wounded, defensive me, and the wiser, openhearted part of me. Rumi also helps me have compassion for the internal, wounded, adolescent Tom, and the current, reactive Tom who wants to lash out in fear and anger. Such understanding and acceptance allows me to get enough distance from the defensiveness so I am not swept away by its demand for self-protection at all costs. From this place, I am able to make choices that better serve me.

How do we learn to handle our responses to the triggering events that life throws at us? First and foremost, we must accept that the feelings that are being triggered are real and are happening in the here and now. Instead of denying feelings, we need to learn how to befriend them. One strategy my patients and students readily respond to is "The Puppy Technique." Think about how we housebreak puppies—with great love and patience. We gently guide them back to the newspaper over and over again, knowing in time they will get it. Occasionally we may feel tired or exasperated, but we know if we're too rough we'll scare the poor things and make it worse. Treat yourself similarly. With great patience and affection, gently yet firmly address the aspects of your responses that need attention, knowing change is not going to happen overnight.

For some people, accepting a difficult situation is almost impossible. They blame themselves for any and all adversities that they encounter. If they were abused as children, for instance, they believe it was their own fault. They go so far as to excuse their abuser's behavior by saying their abusers were victims of their own difficult circumstances. True as that may be, using it to justify the abuser results in my clients' ignoring their feelings of anger and hurt. Instead of holding their abusers accountable, they place any blame for their pain on themselves. The resultant shame keeps some from doing anything to change. For others, shame prevents them from taking credit for anything they do to improve.

Dr. Emmons talks about this phenomenon of self-hatred in our culture. Like me, he has seen many patients who abhor themselves. "It is such a prevalent feeling. It's almost astounding how many people get caught in that belief that they are not okay—that there is something fundamentally wrong with them." While I know it's true (I see it every day in my work), I still can't help but be saddened by the thought of the suffering of countless wounded souls.

How do we become more self-loving? I believe it starts with self-acceptance. When self-deprecating thoughts come up, start by simply noticing them. Berating yourself for berating yourself is not going to help! Accept that you are doing so in this moment and that like everything else, these dark thoughts will pass. Next, treat yourself as you would a good friend. Imagine you were listening to a friend put herself down. How would you respond? Whenever I ask my patients that question, they immediately come up with compassionate replies—after all, they know what suffering is all about. They definitely would not be judgmental and say things like "you're exaggerating" or blame their friend by saying "it's your fault, you always do this." Instead, they tell me they would remind her of her good qualities. Some even go so far as to say they would tell her they love her. Why don't we treat ourselves the same way?

Until we can accept who we are, we can't make the deep, lasting change we seek. I have found that for many people it is hard to stick to a diet or an exercise routine, for example, because they hate themselves for being overweight or out of shape. Those negative feelings may goad us toward initiating a change, but change undertaken by goading rarely lasts. The underlying belief that we are bad seems to derail efforts to improve ourselves. When efforts to change come from love and self-acceptance, however, we are far more likely to stick to the plan. As Dr. Emmons says, it is a paradox that in order to change, we have to accept where we are right now, love handles and all. I find the same thing with my coaching and psychotherapy clients—and in myself. Lasting change only occurs from a place of self-acceptance.

Based on research and his work with thousands of patients, Dr. Emmons has discovered several tools to help foster self-acceptance. For starters, he suggests that we build in time during the day to let our minds settle down and let go of all the distractions that keep us from being in the moment. There is an added blessing when we let our minds relax. Dr. Emmons explains that when you meditate, "you open your mind toward yourself. If you can do that, then you can learn to hold yourself with kindness, to realize that you make mistakes just like everybody else. You're not perfect and nobody is, but that's okay. If you can genuinely have a change of heart toward yourself, then it opens up the possibility of real healing." I call this Full Heart Living.

"The second thing that can open people up to joy is to really be deeply connected to others," Dr. Emmons continues. "I think it is really essential. Being able to love well. It is just a crucial aspect of genuine happiness."

Over the years, in my work as a therapist, I have come to realize that self-love cannot happen in a vacuum. Self-love comes from engagement in "community." Whether that community is comprised of a spouse, a lover, friends, siblings or other family members, or a combination, we're social beings. Loving others—and being loved by others—feeds the sense of self. (And vice-versa, of course; loving myself helps others love me.)

It's true, there are times when I am embarrassed at my own inability to practice what I preach. Here I am, writing a book on happiness, in which one of the main tenets is that connecting with others brings happiness. Yet at times I can't seem to manage to connect with my own friends and family. At times, I am reactive. In other words, much of what I do is in direct response to the actions of others. Reactive is a term that comes from chemistry. Many chemicals become reactive when mixed with other chemicals. A person who is reactive does things in response to others. For example, I get miserable when my husband doesn't respond to me in the way I need him to. When he seems not to hear me, I withdraw.

I believe one of the most important things we can do as healers is face our own demons. As Iyanla Vanzant says, "Your willingness to look at your darkness is what empowers you to change." I must accept my tendency toward reactivity so when I perceive that I am being unfairly judged or dismissed, I do not have to lash out or withdraw. I can make different choices. Using the tools we've talked about in this book, especially mindfulness, I can acknowledge when anger and the urge to withdraw arise, and go toward myself and my suffering, instead of running away from them. For this to happen, I first have to acknowledge what is happening, accept that it has occurred, and then take some deep breaths and center my mind. I focus on letting go of all the reactive thoughts screaming in my head. I acknowledge and accept that *I am not perfect, that I am just a struggling soul like everyone else. I can still love myself and be imperfect.*

One of the things that most helped me do so was a workshop for psychotherapists I attended on The Power of Mindfulness, with Ronald D. Siegel, Psy.D. One of the things I heard him say is that the process of psychotherapy naturally increases one's awareness of thought patterns. While that may seem like a no-brainer, like a lightning bolt, his next sentence jolted me: "We're actually less nuts, but we notice more craziness because we're more refined."

Those wise words have come into my mind often since. Helping others examine their irrational thinking in my work prompts me to assess mine (and vice versa, of course—as healers, we must do our own work so that we can help our clients). So I may not have more crazy thoughts than others. I just notice them more. What a relief! I'm accepting myself more. Yup, I sometimes experience irrational thoughts, I now think. I also have way more rational ones, thank God.

As Dr. Emmons says, "We need to really begin with our mind. We begin with allowing the mind to calm down at least a little bit so that we can be aware of our experiences, our thoughts and emotional reactions. If we're aware of them, we can choose what we do with them."

Whenever I notice my reactivity is getting out of hand, I recommit to daily meditation and to self-care, including adequate downtime so I am not overwhelmed. I also recommit to treating those who upset me with kindness, no matter how frustrated I am. I pledge to be more forthcoming when disagreements arise.

But Dr. Emmons goes on to say, "What really determines whether we end up feeling happy or not is how we respond to [the events in our lives]. It's what we do given the things that happen to us. That's what really makes the difference, I think. How we handle it. How we perceive what's happening to us."

I think of Tracy stumbling across chalk-written words on the Chicago sidewalk (described in Chapter 2: Defining happiness), which transformed his day: "Today is an opportunity."

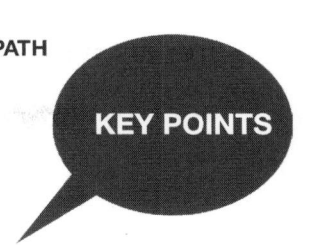

KEY POINTS

- While suffering may be unavoidable, joy is equally possible
- Happier people are self-accepting; they embrace the fullness of themselves, including those parts that are imperfect
- Self-acceptance allows us to love ourselves and others more deeply
- Settling the mind, opening the heart, and connecting with others all contribute to self acceptance
- It's not so much what happens to us that determines our happiness as how we respond to those events
- Loving others—and being loved by others—feeds our sense of self
- Loving yourself helps others love you, and loving yourself helps you love others more

PUTTING IT INTO PRACTICE

EVERY DAY, FIND TIME TO SETTLE DOWN YOUR MIND Do five minutes of breathing. Meditate for 20 minutes. Take a mindful walk; with each step repeat a self-affirmation. If you are religious, recommit to your faith and start a daily habit of prayer. Breathe. Practice patience and mindfulness. See Chapter 6: Developing mindfulness, for ideas on this.

INTERRUPT EMOTIONAL HIGH-JACKING When your mind is scattered or racing, interrupt the flow by attending to the breath, the body, or objects.

> **PRACTICE "SQUARE" BREATHING** Breathe in to a count of eight, hold to a count of eight, breathe out to a count of eight, hold for a count of eight. Complete the cycle a total of eight times.

NEAR AND FAR Look at something far away. Really notice what you see. Now examine an object very near. Bring your full attention to the task.

HUM, WHISTLE, OR BREATHE THROUGH A STRAW.

MIND-BODY PRACTICES such as Yoga, Qi Gong, and Tai Chi are very effective for getting us out of our heads.

EMBRACE THE PARADOX We need to accept who we are and change behaviors that aren't serving us.

ACCEPT that just like everyone, you make mistakes. You're as human as the next guy. Have you ever examined an Amish quilt? Look closely enough, and you'll find an imperfection. It's included purposely as a reminder that only the Creator is—and creates things that are—perfect. I love that idea! I'm even practcing it in this book. See if you can find the intentional error in this paragraph.

WRITE IT OUT Keep a journal of when your demons show up. Is there a pattern to the time or day when they become especially active? Is there a particular person or place that triggers them? It might be good to avoid these triggers until you have learned how to quiet your mind.

CONNECT with others. See Chapter 9: Connecting, for many ideas on this.

Connecting:
All you need is love

The stand-out message I got from all the people I spoke to about happiness is how relationships are crucial not just to having, but to maintaining genuine happiness. As Dr. Emmons explains so eloquently, "We are wired to be connected with others. It is built in to us—our whole being. I think that is one of the biggest turning points, even in someone who's depressed, is to be able to connect in more meaningful ways with others. Cultivating a good heart and really creating deep connections with others and with yourself is just crucial for genuine happiness." I feel a tremor arise in my whole being as I hear Dr. Emmons express this.

What does cultivating a good heart and creating deep connections look like? In short, cultivating a good heart means being kind, and treating others as we would like to be treated. Good-hearted folks express keen interest in others, asking questions about what matters to them and listening deeply. They treat others with respect. They are free of judgment; they allow others to hold differing opinions and positions. They accept people for who they are.

ONLY ONE HAPPINESS

"There is only one happiness in life, to love and be loved."
  ~George Sand

If cultivating a good heart is how we establish good relationships, then knowing how to connect on a deep level is how we preserve and enhance them. We deepen connections by being "real" with others, taking risks, and exposing our more vulnerable sides, rather than hiding parts of ourselves we deem less-than-perfect. It also means investing time in relationships and taking the initiative to maintain contact.

AVOID DEATHBED REGRETS

Barry becomes serious as he recalls the words of a friend who was terminally ill. "Before she passed, she said, 'You know, now that I'm dying, I have not laid here thinking, 'Oh, I wish I had gotten my paperwork done faster. I am laying here wondering why I didn't take care of some of those friendships better.'" I feel his sadness.

"So, when it comes down to what's really important," Barry continues, "it's going to be our relationships. It's not, I need to get my paperwork done. Who gives a shit? If it comes down to work or relationships, I'm going with relationships. So many things are relational. So when relationships go well, I seem to be happier. So, I attend to them. They're important to me."

Right Relationship and Being Present

I feel as though she is letting me in on a profound secret, when, during my video interview with her, therapist Mia touches upon the subject of relationships. "I feel really blessed that I have more love in my life than most people I know. And I know we don't brag in Minnesota, and I'm not bragging. I'm just telling you that. I think it's true." Knowing Mia, I can vouch for her humility. Having experienced her openheartedness, I find it easy to believe she is very loved.

"So I've spent my life learning how to be in Right Relationship," Mia proceeds. Here, Mia highlights a crucial element in many Buddhist teachings (although it also appears in Quaker, Christian, and perhaps other religious material as well as in many Native teachings). Right Relationship involves interacting in a manner that is respectful to all and aids the common good. Take note of the first part, "respectful to all." Something that many of my coaching and psychotherapy clients forget is that "all" also includes themselves. Yes, we are called to be respectful, kind, helpful, and openhearted with others. We also need to do so with ourselves. A friend's recent Facebook post sums up this concept nicely: "Do no harm but take no shit." In Right Relationship, we treat others and ourselves well.

Mia dedicates her life to the most important thing: building Right Relationship. What's more important than connecting well, treating others and ourselves with respect and kindness? No wonder she's so happy.

I ask Mia how we create loving relationships.

"I think for me creating loving relationships has a lot to do with how we make contact," Mia tells me. Her features remain soft, but her voice is so clear and strong that I almost have chills. She is convinced, and convincing. "And by contact I mean being present," she continues. "People respond so much better when you are really present with them. They love it."

"Can you give an example?" I ask.

Mia barely needs to think. "I have this really dear friend, Dave, and we go to Twins games together. We went to the brat stand and I got our brats. And he said, 'Wow, you just totally made that person's day,'" referring to the vendor.

Mia looks to the side, as though she's replaying the scene in her mind. She tells me that Dave continued, "Did you notice that nobody else looked her in the eye? Nobody else said, 'Hey, how are you doing?'"

Mia pauses. "Dave was right. I had looked her in the eye, and I had smiled, and I had asked her how she was doing. And I meant everything I said, and she felt that. So she and I just had this really brief exchange."

Mia continues, "Because I am quite loving, and I am happy to extend this love, it feels really natural to me. I feel like I just want to be with people and really appreciate what they're doing."

I add, "Even if it's 'just' the person at the hot dog counter?"

"Yes. Especially the person at the counter, because that's a lot of what our life is filled with. The person at the counter matters, and small exchanges matter." Mia is so emphatic here, I suspect, because whether it's the brat seller, the dry cleaner, or the person next to us at the bus stop, so much of modern life is spent in contact with relative strangers. Also, whenever we truly connect with anyone, no matter how briefly, our best self emerges, and we enrich the other and ourselves.

Mia walks the talk. I love meeting her for coffee, which we do every now and then. She listens deeply when I talk about something, asks discerning questions, and makes astute comments. All serve to make me feel valued. She also tells me about what is going on with her in complete honesty and openness. By telling me about herself, I feel trusted. She embodies the presence of which she speaks. I am convinced that being present like this brings out the best in ourselves and the best in others. It is what makes our relationships flourish.

ASK QUESTIONS

Want a simple way of deepening your relationships? One of the easiest yet too often overlooked ways involves expressing interest in others. From his warm Connecticut living room, Barry touches on this idea when he reflects on his partner, Tom. In groups, Tom tends to be on the quiet side. "I notice him being much more pleased with our company when somebody's asking him about himself. A lot of people don't. Most people talk about themselves. Ask questions. I think that's a very caring thing to do."

Relationships Take Work

While it's no surprise that everyone I interview agrees good relationships are essential to happiness, what might be astonishing is how much trouble we get into with those closest to us. I've come to wonder if the universe conspires to place us with loved ones who unconsciously bring out our best and worst. Sometimes we're delighted to discover how kind and giving we are. Other times we're shocked and embarrassed by how selfish and mean we can be. For some people, the reverse might be true. These folks already know what stinkers they can be, but give them say a grandchild or two, and suddenly they're as kind and giving as can be. Close relationships of all kinds provide opportunities to recognize our true, full selves, including the parts we're proudest and most ashamed of. I suspect those closest to us, with their stable presence and more or less unconditional love, provide the safety we need to expose these more vulnerable—sometimes called the "shadow"—sides, whether loving, spiteful, or a combination of the two.

When we can be more fully ourselves—including all those parts of us that people admire and the parts we often aim to hide—and still be accepted by others and by ourselves, we heal. To me, becoming whole in this way, embracing the totality of our being, is what it means to heal. Not that we necessarily act on all our impulses, mind you, but that we embrace the fact that we have the impulses themselves. While it may seem counter-intuitive to some, doing so reduces the chance that we'll act rashly.

By embracing all of our potential, the good the bad and the ugly, we become whole. To do so, we must bring our shadow into the light—to expose it. Being in close relationships with others allows and invites this to happen. One of two things tends to happen when we deny parts of ourselves. We project the unwanted part outward, seeing evil in others, or we unconsciously despise ourselves. Suffering inevitably results, as we either hate others or ourselves. When we are more integrated and accept-ing of our full selves, we are free of such projections, which provides the opportunity to be happier.

I know firsthand how easy it is for shadows to come out and test rela-tionships. My shadow emerged in spades when I was about to turn 50. During a two-hour drive for a weekend getaway with my spouse, Greg, I wanted to explore plans and share feelings about my upcoming birthday party. Tackling projects together and sharing feelings are essential compo-nents of good relationships, strengthening bonds and creating goodwill.

MAKING RELATIONSHIPS WORK AT WORK

One of my interviewees, Barry, was the director of a large college counseling center in Connecticut. When I ask him what makes for good relations at work, he tells me this story about one of his therapists who was "a curmudgeon with a 'K.' Not only does he think the glass is half empty, he's put out about the damn glass."

When it came time for this employee's annual performance review, Barry was honest. "He's a very good therapist, and he's a workhorse. He puts out the numbers. I like this guy. But there was a problem. He was too negative around his colleagues. I said to him, 'You know what, you could be the most talented person here, and if nobody likes you, you might as well not be good at anything.' To be successful, you have to manage your interpersonal relationships and be thoughtful about that."

I ask Barry to explain how to go about being supportive and encouraging. "Facilitating folks," he explains, "thanking folks, and sort of being very thoughtful about the interpersonal relations."

Barry tells me attending to work relationships honors the process—focusing on how the work gets done, not just the desired outcome. It starts with getting to know coworkers, expressing genuine interest in them personally, and listening deeply. Saying thank you and providing recognition, it also involves valuing their contributions. Good conflict management, where both sides are heard and validated and compromises are mutually agreed upon, is another key ingredient.

When colleagues feel heard and valued, when they experience an environment of mutual respect, Barry says, they feel safe and appreciated. And when they do, they are likely to produce better results and feel good about how it all gets done. Then they're motivated to do even more.

I had been thinking about how to mark the milestone of my 50th birthday for more than a year, and Greg and I had yet to talk about it in detail. The big day was three months away, and the plans I had been making in my head were getting complicated. I preferred the party take place in our home, and I wanted the centerpiece to be a birthday ritual in which a facilitator guides friends and family in expressing their feelings about the birthday person. It's like a eulogy without having to die! I thought I'd invite a select group of 20 to the ritual, and ask 30 friends to come afterward. (Fifty friends for 50 years, get it?!) All 50 would enjoy dinner, live music, a sing-along, fireworks, and s'mores. I wanted Greg to share my enthusiasm and to get his input on and help with some of the details. What better time to do so than on a long drive.

Two of my favorite questions are *What if?* and *How could we make it so?* What foods do we serve? How many people? Who could we ask to play piano? What about beverages? Such questions make me feel energized and excited, and I find exploring options with open-minded, openhearted abandon connects people and allows innovative options to unfold.

I pull out several catering menus and begin the conversation. With my usual, "what about this, what about that?" I tell him about wanting to have the ritual when I hear the first sigh. Then his questions and criticism begin:

"How many people total? You need a big tent outside."

"No room in the yard for a tent? Then have it somewhere else."

"If it's at our home, don't invite so many people."

"What's the budget?"

"Why not just do it like my 50th birthday and have a bowling party?"

Stunned and stung, I don't reply. I don't even know what to say. The conversation has devolved from "sharing and connecting" to definitions of fairness and financial terms. Now I let out a sigh. I realize just how fully I have not been heard; Greg is not picking up on what I want. Worse, I feel undermined and that my ideas are dumb, unfair, and apparently too expensive. I close my manila folder along with a bit of my heart. I shut down. This is my worst side coming out—the petulant child who punishes with silence.

A month passes. I continue practicing my happiness program, but I'm sad and frustrated. My program feels anemic because I don't feel connected to Greg. I recognize that I need to address this situation with him, but I am not sure how.

As we're dressing for brunch with our neighbors, I realize that my chance to clear the air has come. I decide to tell Greg how I feel. Not realizing the level of my irritation, however, and therefore failing to calm myself before speaking, I come across far too abrasively. "When we talk about the party, I need your 100 percent support." My volume rises and I stare at him—hard. "I don't want you undermining, criticizing, or judging me. I need you to help figure out how to make things happen, not tell me my ideas are unreasonable or unattainable."

I take Greg's silence to mean he understands that he was too abrupt when we talked about it in the car last month. It doesn't yet hit me that I'd come on too strongly. As Greg is preparing eggs for the brunch, he tells me he feels I have blamed and shamed him.

At my limit, with my resentment reaching critical mass, I lash out. "What are you talking about?" I screech. "I shamed you? You shamed me when I tried to talk about it on the car ride. I'm trying to tell you I need your support. Don't miss my message because my delivery was harsh." We drop the discussion.

Unfortunately it's not over. For several days I can't seem to get our argument out of my mind. I am so furious, I barely talk to him. When I withdraw like this, Greg gets anxious. Understandably, he feels rejected, which triggers unrealistic worries in him. To his credit, Greg suggests we try a "PR/CD," or Personal Reflection/Couple Dialogue, a technique we learned at Heart-to-Heart, an intensive couples' retreat and support group we attended a few years prior.

For more information on Heart-to-Heart Retreats, visit http://heart.mn.cx/h2h_what-happens.htm

PERSONAL REFLECTION/COUPLES DIALOGUE (PR/CD)

While it's best to learn and practice the Personal Reflection/ Couples Dialogue (PR/CD) process from an experienced couple at a Heart-to-Heart Retreat, here's an introduction. A PR/CD involves three steps. The couple agrees to write on a specific topic in response to a series of one to three open-ended questions.

An example topic might be Finances. Questions might include
a.) What financial issues do we avoid discussing?
b.) How does this impact our relationship?
1) Identify the topic.
2) Select one to three relevant, open-ended questions.
3) Both partners write simultaneously for 20 minutes to identical questions.
4) Simultaneously, each then silently reads twice what the other has written—once with the heart and once with the head.
5) For 20 minutes, the couple engages in a respectful conversation. Each listens deeply, speaks mindfully, avoids using blaming or shaming language, accepts responsibility for her/his part, and assertively states needs and wants.

The beauty of the PR/CD is that writing and reading of each partner's words tends to create enough distance from the problems so that the couple can talk through things calmly, without becoming emotionally triggered.

While the topic is usually more contained, we chose to write about our recent experiences with one another generally. I write: "I tried to tell you what I needed, but experienced you as critical, exasperated, and frustrated about planning my party or if I disagree with you. I wish I didn't have to tell you this, but I'd like to not be belittled and made to feel that

I am wrong for wanting things to be the way I want them to be. The message I get is that what I want is unreasonable, unachievable—and that I am stupid."

As Greg silently reads my words, his brow furrows and the corners of his mouth drop. "I'm sorry," he says. "I'm shocked I was coming across so rigidly. I was just trying to be helpful."

Greg writes: "I wish we could disagree or get angry sometimes and still stay connected to each other and resolve the issue. I know that I am at least half of the negative dynamic. I really want to change this because I hate not being connected. I'm sorry that I wasn't better able to take in your message about the party. Your tone should have been my clue that I'm really not supporting you. Instead I just heard shaming words. I should have looked deeper at what you were meaning—instead of the exact words. I am excited for your party and want to be involved and help. I'm proud of you for celebrating this milestone—and need to keep my judgments to myself unless you ask."

Reading Greg's words calms me. He saw how our behavior was distancing us from one another. With his role in our rift acknowledged, I feel understood and supported; it's as though I can safely get back "in" our relationship. From there, I'm able to take responsibility for my part. I realize I'm as much to blame as Greg. I failed to tell him right away how unsupported I was feeling, and withholding such powerful feelings created a barrier between us. When at last I did tell him, I was too aggressive. When I didn't like his response, I gave him the silent treatment, which to him feels cruel. I feel bad that I was so mean, and I regret that I'd been holding so much back.

For both of us to be happier in our relationship, I need not only to ask him to examine how he communicates, but to also make an effort to communicate better myself. I must check things out within myself when I'm feeling unheard or frustrated. I need to practice what I preach, which is to accept what's arising in myself and in our relationship, and assert-ively express what I need. In many situations, I am masterful at doing so. Under the right conditions, however, I revert back to old patterns. Poor

Greg got caught up in a perfect storm of my feelings, and I let him have it with my old passive-aggressive habits.

Having a conflict and successfully working through it—being fully present with and accepting of one another, acknowledging the truth of our shadows and coming through it maintaining our love and respect for one another—made us a stronger, better team and helped me feel better about myself.

While I wouldn't wish a misunderstanding like this on anyone, in retrospect I can honestly say I'm glad we went through it. The experience provided an opportunity to see our shadows and related habits, and to change. It's an example of what psychologist and researcher John Gottman (author of *The Relationship Cure* and *The Seven Principles for Making Marriage Work*) calls rupture and repair. No intimate relationship is free of conflict. Couples that stay together, Gottman (who I think of as a modern day relationship guru) says, become masters at repairing any ruptures in their connection. Greg and I were able to navigate a sticky situation and come out stronger.

As for the 50th birthday party? It turned out just as I had hoped. It was at our home, replete with a beautiful, heart-warming ritual, fireworks, sing-along, live music, and s'mores. The best part, though, was being with family and friends, strengthening and celebrating our connections.

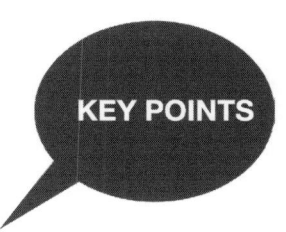

KEY POINTS

- Everyone I interviewed identified relationships as a key component in their happiness; they all actively develop and maintain connections with others
- Being fully present—eliminating distractions, smiling, making eye contact, and deep listening—fosters connections

- Close relationships provide opportunities to recognize our true, full selves, including parts that we're proud of and ashamed of
- With their stable presence and unconditional love, those closest to us provide the safety to expose these more vulnerable—sometimes called the "shadow"—sides
- In functional relationships, it's essential to embrace our shadow and take responsibility for our part in conflict
- Small kindnesses, such as simply smiling or saying hello, can make a profound impact
- When conflict arises, the key is to repair any rupture in connection

PUTTING IT INTO PRACTICE

REACH OUT Contact friends with whom you've been out of touch. Ask a coworker to lunch. Send a family member a card. Stop by your elderly neighbor's place.

TELL PEOPLE YOU CARE ABOUT THEM Some of the most powerful phrases are: I care about you. I'm here for you. I'm here with you. I love you. I'm sorry.

SEEK OUT THE COMPANY OF PEOPLE YOU ADMIRE When I first started in radio, I was amazed how often people agreed to be interviewed. Even when I thought they were too famous or busy, just having the courage to ask often proved fruitful. You don't need a radio show to reach out. Maybe say you're working on a personal project—you! Simply asking markedly increases the probability that they'll say yes. If you don't ask, the answer for sure is no.

INVEST IN THE PEOPLE YOU CARE ABOUT Years ago it occurred to me that relationships are similar to other enterprises. We invest time in our education and our careers, for example. Friendships, too, need time and attention. Think of it as making a deposit in your "Wellbeing

401K." Sometimes I even block off time in my calendar so I'm sure I'll save time for correspondence.

PRACTICE EMOTIONAL INTELLIGENCE Folks with higher EQs (a.k.a. emotional intelligence) have far more satisfying relationships. They tend to be more aware of their own feelings and display more empathy for others'. See *Emotional Intelligence* by Daniel Goleman to get you started. Goleman describes five elements of emotional intelligence and demonstrates how they determine success in relationships, work, and even our physical health.

ASK OTHERS QUESTIONS Demonstrate interest in others by asking their opinions. Inquire about their experiences. Express interest in what they're interested in. When she first sees them, for example, my friend Merra almost always comments on what her friends are wearing. It's like a social appetizer served to warm up the conversational palate. In doing so, Merra tells me (via email) she is "appreciating my friend's beauty and expression—a compliment, enjoying their 'colors'... not so much the clothes themselves." Her friends feel noticed and appreciated, and deeper conversation ensues. Upon meeting a new person at a party, you might gently inquire how they know the host. The response will give you clues about the person's work or hobbies. Ask a follow-up question based on what you learn, and so on.

ENCOURAGE When you notice people doing something well, tell them.

SUPPORT If someone seems in need, offer help. Be specific. "I'd be glad to watch the kids while you go to your doctor's appointment" is better than, "Let me know if there's anything I can do to help."

ALLOW OTHERS TO NOTICE AND LOVE YOU Too often, my clients complain that others don't approach them. After careful examination, however, it often becomes clear that the client isn't noticing others' "bids" for connection. Failing to maintain eye contact, for example, or not returning others' smiles turns people off. Without sacrificing personal safety, of course, be open to others who may be subtly cueing you that they'd like to connect. See John Gottman's book *The Relationship Cure,* which introduces the concept of the "emotional bid," the fundamental unit of emotional connection. Gottman outlines a five-step, research-based, time-tested approach for improving relationships of all kinds.

REALLY SEE THE OTHER Even the cashier, teller, or tollbooth atten-dant. Make eye contact. Engage with a warm hello. Ask how their day is going—and truly listen to the answer. Notice how you feel.

When in conflict, **CHECK IT OUT**. Make sure you understand what the other is saying before responding.

Still in conflict? **TRY A SOFT START-UP.** Yes, it's important for you to be assertive and state what you feel and need. Tone of voice makes all the difference. Speaking calmly and with a neutral look on your face will get you much further than yelling and scowling.

ASSESS YOUR FRIENDSHIPS
As Philip does, take a look at those you spend time with.
- Do these people inspire you?
- Do they bring out the best in you?
- Do they challenge you?

BE GOLDEN Treat others as you would like to be treated. It is the Golden Rule, after all. It's golden for a reason.

BE KIND To me, being kind is probably the most important thing of all.

CHAPTER 10

Bouncing back with resilience: 10,000 joys, 10,000 sorrows

While it might be tempting to believe that happier people have fewer difficulties and challenges, there's no evidence of that. In fact, having heard the stories of my interview subjects and my happier patients, I have found that happy people experience just as many unhappy encounters with the world as anyone. The difference is in how they face them.

The story of my friend Nancy and how she coped with adversity still resonates with me. She provides a profound, yet hopeful example of what can happen when life hits you hard. She and I are sitting in my living room having tea. We are talking about when we first met, some 14 years ago, when she and I were at an intensive workshop for psychotherapists who practice couples therapy. Over lunch on the last day of the workshop Nancy shared with me the story of her own relationship. Nancy was 18 years into what she thought was a happy marriage. She and her husband were just beginning to enjoy their beautiful, new, years-in-the-making dream house. They had meticulously designed every detail and oversaw it being built from the ground up the year before.

Nancy appears pensive as she recalls a beautiful afternoon just before her world fell apart. She was driving home under a cloudless blue sky, with the sun casting golden rays through her neighborhood's tree-lined streets. "I remember looking around at how wonderful everything seemed," Nancy sighs, recalling this stellar moment now many years past. She remembers that she actually told herself, "I have this really good life." She hesitates.

"I was glad I took the moment to notice how beautiful it all looked," Nancy says. Her features drop as she tells me what came next. A few days later, out of the blue, her husband told her he had made a unilateral decision. "He said: 'I don't want to be married anymore, and I don't want to work on it.'"

Nancy felt as though her world had fallen apart, and in a way, it had. Without a hint of warning, she not only lost her marriage, but also her life-partner, lover, and best friend. "It was like a truck hit me," Nancy recalls, looking down at her cup of tea. "The worst part was that he absolutely did not want to work on it." Nancy grimaces. "I'd never considered that someone wouldn't want to work on his or her marriage," she says, shaking her head. After her husband dropped this bomb, Nancy experienced "everything people who grieve go through: the unreality of it, the shock, the trauma. It was unbelievable. My life as I'd known it was over." Her husband had blown up their marriage. What Nancy didn't realize at the time was that he had blown her up, as well. "I didn't know who I was anymore. Everything I knew was now different. Suddenly, I'm not who I used to be, and I could not imagine how this would ever get better."

Unfortunately, another bomb exploded. "I was already feeling there must be something wrong with me that my husband would leave me," Nancy tells me, when she found out her husband had been seeing another woman. The affair had begun four months before he told Nancy he was leaving. This latest news was soul-crushing. "Now there's someone he likes better. The feeling that there is something wrong with me was even more pronounced."

At times like these, we are sometimes mysteriously "directed" to just the right book. This proved true in Nancy's case when she encountered *The Journey from Abandonment to Healing* by Susan Anderson. "It was especially useful. It helped me understand the physiological responses I was going through, that being around him was almost a terrifying experience. The book normalized that when going through a betrayal like that, the person who had been your protector, confidante, and best friend can feel like a predator. Even being around him would put my body into this huge anxiety and terror, really. It helped to know this is a normal response to betrayal." That was a huge revelation.

A friend recommended a support group for people going through separation and divorce, and Nancy, not without some reluctance, attended. "I remember how I was there, just telling my story. I could hardly get through it without just sobbing and sobbing. And everybody else who was there was crying when they talked. I remember being comforted by that. But then when I was leaving, thinking, 'I don't want to be in this club. This is not the club I want to belong to.'" She shakes her head at the memory, adding, "But I belong to it."

A silver lining was the long-lasting friendships she ended up forming from that very support group. Despite the diversity of those present, "these people became friends. Fourteen years later, we're still friends. They're people I never would have met otherwise, people who were in completely different worlds. An artist, a professor, an HR person in a major corporation—people I wouldn't typically run into. We came together around this loss, and we're now good friends. That was a real gift. We still get together and refer to it," Nancy continues, "it" meaning their common loss, "which is very useful. Because we recognize all that pain we each have gone through to get to this point." Nancy is referring to the healing power of having our pain validated by someone we trust because they've endured a similar loss. The sense of validation may go even deeper and be enhanced by the reciprocity. The other has contributed to our healing and we have contributed to theirs.

Appearing to collect herself, Nancy pauses. Then another memory strikes. She looks down. "There was a moment where the pain of it was so great that I remember waking up, and my heart felt like it was being literally ripped. I felt this tear such that I just cried out. It was a physical tear. I cried out with the agony of it, not understating how could it be that hard, how could it be that painful."

She breathes. "The experience was devastating," Nancy continues after a moment. "The anger, the terror, the loss, the 'I can't believe this is happening,' the 'I don't know who I am,' all of that just was my reality for a long time. Not months. More like years."

I ask what helped her endure and cope. Nancy's features brighten slightly as she replies, "People kept telling me, 'the most important thing you can do right now is take care of yourself.' And I took that to heart." She tells me how she had lost her appetite and begun to rapidly lose weight. Having always been fit and naturally lean, Nancy did not need to shed any pounds. "The first thing I had to do was figure out how to eat so I wouldn't lose all my strength," she tells me, a note of determination returning to her voice. She decided to buy healthy, prepared meals and keep them in her fridge or freezer. At mealtime, all she had to do was heat them up.

Nancy added other restorative practices to her self-care. She got a massage every week, started yoga and meditation, and increased her regular gym exercise routine. Most important, she made sure to spend time with friends so she wouldn't isolate. In short, she made herself her top priority. This is key because taking care of ourselves can spell the difference between overcoming a crisis or staying in it. We have to make a conscious decision to take care of ourselves to make it through life's challenges (see Chapter 4: Establishing a foundation, for more on this).

An avid reader, Nancy turned to reading spiritual books, especially the writings of Buddhist nun Pema Chodron, who had also suffered a wrenching divorce. "Her books were probably my most important inspirational lifeline," Nancy says, "because she talked about being with what is. She talked about impermanence. She talked about how to be in the moment, being present. When you're grieving like that, the past and the future are just agonizing, because the past is full of these memories, first the good ones and then the really, really awful ones, that you could relive over and over again. But there comes a point where you wonder, 'How do I get to this moment and not worry about the future, because I don't know what that's going to be? I'm not who I used to be, and I'm not who

I'm going to be.' So practicing being in the moment became life saving. I would get into the shower and feel the hot water on my skin, and it would bring me into the present moment."

I am stunned at the depth of Nancy's pain—and her insightful story of recovery. We all know people who have gone through great losses, but we rarely get to hear the inside story, the real nuts and bolts. "This was the beginning of recovering and finding my new self," Nancy adds, her gentle voice now strong and sure. "There is something about 'growing up,'" Nancy continues, as she begins to bring it all together, "to the reality of what life is. There is no promise, there's no guarantee, there isn't the 'if I'm good then I'll get this reward, or God's going to take care of me.' The only person who can take care of me is me. Other people can support me and remind me that I'm worth taking care of. But I still have to be the one to do it. To grow up to the reality that there's no guarantee somebody is going to be with me forever, that I'm going to have my dream house forever. I got those things." She looks out my dining room window, where a gentle breeze stirs the leaves of the neighbor's dogwoods.

Nancy turns to me and reveals the real hard truth of her ordeal. "When we go through grief and welcome it, when we're willing to show up to grief and the pain of it, there is a maturing that happens about life. There are beautiful things and really, really hard things. They will come again. The really hard things will come again. What I came out of it was knowing I developed a set of skills that were invaluable, and I rely on them all the time."

A source of great joy in Nancy's life now is her work. About two years after her husband left, a friend told her about a job opening at a local hospice. Nancy instantly felt, without a shred of doubt, that she could do the job. "I know this," she found herself saying. In time, that job led to her finding her true calling as a grief counselor.

"I felt like it was fate," she says, especially since after the divorce she was uncertain about what she wanted to do professionally. She had been a psychotherapist in private practice for decades. With the grief work, everything clicked. She had the background as a psychotherapist, and now "I could bring to other people the support that I'd had. Now I could offer it to others."

Nancy was determined that her loss wouldn't be in vain. "There's no getting over your loss, but there is getting through it. And if I'm going to come through it, I want to come out with something. I want there to be something on the other side of this that will be useful." Her work provides just that.

And then Nancy adds something that surprised me, and thoroughly impressed me with its heartfelt honesty. "I miss to this day my family life—the dream that I had," Nancy acknowledges. "I miss that. I wish there had been some way I could have had that. But I would not trade who I am now and what I gained from this. If somebody said you could have the life you had, or you can have who you are now. I could never go back. I would never choose that. My life is a treasure. I still have sadness, and I still have pain, and I still miss what might have become. But who I've become is solid. It's substantial. I know who I am. I wasn't always sure before, but I know who I am. I don't wake up happy every day, but I do wake up with gratitude." I marvel that Nancy is able to acknowledge that she still misses her old life. Most people never reveal this very human side of recovery: while the pain may lessen, the loss remains.

My tea, long since forgotten, sits cold in its mug. I breathe deeply and drink in Nancy with my eyes. Then she turns to me and says, "There's one more thing I should add that was important to my healing," she says. "I made a decision to not demonize my husband. He had a story, too. He was a struggling human being." She knew holding onto resentment would harm her, and she was right. By not turning her husband into "the bad guy," she spared turning herself into a victim.

In enduring this ordeal, Nancy provides a phenomenal example of the power of resilience. Instead of denying and avoiding her experiences and all the attendant emotions, she courageously embraced them. Supporting herself, and surrounding herself with those who supported her, in time she bounced back from adversity and became a better, stronger person. In the process, she found a new community, a new life's work, and a new self.

10,000 Joys, 10,000 Sorrows

I find Nancy's story mesmerizing; it's as though I have witnessed a complete transformation of a person. I am reminded of a story Dr. Emmons shares. A woman from the audience approached him after he gave a public lecture. "She wanted to thank me for my book *The Chemistry of Joy*," Dr. Emmons tells me. "Her story was that she had lost her daughter a few years ago. The young girl had a terminal illness and was not expected to live long. After a few years, her daughter died as expected. Naturally, the mom was devastated. She was anguished about the loss even though it was expected. It was still a huge loss, and she became depressed. It took her a long time—a couple of years—to get out of that depression." She told Dr. Emmons that what saved her was reading *The Chemistry of Joy*. Dr. Emmons looks wistful.

I ask why he thinks she found it so illuminating. "My sense is that she re-oriented her focus to the joy that she got from her daughter's presence while she was alive, and that helped her tap into gratitude for having her in her life for as many years as she did. I believe she must have experienced what I emphasized in my book—using your attention to create higher inner states like gratitude, compassion, and generosity through attention and repetition," says Dr. Emmons. I gasp; enduring the loss of a child? It's one of the hardest things I can imagine. How does one find gratitude in anything after that, let alone generosity or compassion?

"It's not that she didn't feel that loss or didn't acknowledge it," Dr. Emmons explains. "She still grieved over it. But she was able to carry both of those things at the same time." In other words, she could feel the loss *and* the joy. Pairing up joy with grief is unusual, but like any other paradox, it can be revealing. "I think this is a very authentic way of talking about joy," says Dr. Emmons. "Joy is not a feeling," he elaborates, "nor is it something that is dependent upon circumstances. It is always there even if we are carrying in one hand some kind of pain, illness, sorrow, or loss, and in the other hand it is very possible for us to be carrying this sense of affirmity, peacefulness, connectedness."

To illuminate further, Dr. Emmons adds, "The Buddhists have a great phrase for this. They talk about the 10,000 joys and the 10,000 sorrows, the idea being that in a given lifetime we have about an equal amount of both."

Listening to Dr. Emmons, I feel as though I am finally getting key information I have needed my entire life. As human beings, it's natural for us to only want those 10,000 joys. But there's just no avoiding the sorrowful or the difficult side of life.

An essential part of resilience is facing pain bravely and learning to manage those hard transitions from grief to acceptance. Like Nancy, we all need to remember that there are no guarantees in life. The only thing we have in our power is to learn how to be ready if and when sorrow comes. Nancy's story also reveals just how important self-care (eating right, exercising, meditating, being with friends) is to recovery.

ACKNOWLEDGING TRANSITIONS

Small acts can help us make conscious transitions, be they good or bad. In graduate school, I learned a simple exercise that fosters acknowledging all sides of transitions. My family adopted it when our son, Elliot, was young. This ritual helped us ease the transition back to everyday life after vacations. On the way home, the three of us reviewed all the things we loved about the trip. Our son might say spending time with his cousins and his Uncle Joe, I'd say eating at my favorite childhood restaurant or seeing my folks. We'd then list what we were looking forward to upon returning home, such as seeing the dog or sleeping in our own beds. We might also acknowledge what we won't miss or what we aren't looking forward to when we get back home, such as going back to school or starting up a difficult project. The act of verbally acknowledging these truths is one way to honor the passing from one stage into another.

"What really decides whether we end up feeling happy or not," Dr. Emmons explains, "is how we respond to [our sorrows]. It's what we do given the things that happen to us." In his calm, open, reassuring manner, he adds, "We are given a certain set of things that we bring into this life, and how then do we respond to that? What do we do in relation to the challenging things, the stressful things that occur in our lives?" I couldn't agree more. What really makes a difference is not what occurs to us, but how we handle it, how we bounce back from adversity. Dr. Emmons is referring, of course, to resilience.

"There is a lot Within our Power to Keep Feeding Resilience"

I always want to know more about resilience, and how we can develop and maintain it. Getting excited, I ask Dr. Emmons to elaborate.

Dr. Emmons says resilience is the ability to experience whatever life throws our way yet "not become overly depressed or overly anxious or sick in some other way." He uses this great water cooler metaphor that I often think about. I ask him to share it. "If you imagine a water cooler—like the one in a typical busy office—now imagine such a container residing deep inside your body. Next, imagine that this cooler doesn't contain water but instead is filled with an elixir that keeps you healthy and able to respond to stressful things while still retaining a sense of balance." Too much stress, lack of sleep, poor nutrition, or not enough exercise, for example, drains the elixir from your cooler. The result is that you become depleted, leading or contributing to "depression, anxiety, or some other illness."

The key is to keep your cooler sufficiently filled so it won't become too low. "If you're doing the things that keep feeding and supplying that elixir, then you will not become ill," Dr. Emmons says. Maintaining the elixir can help ward off everything from anxiety and depression to colds and flu bugs. "I find that an empowering way of thinking," Dr. Emmons continues. "There is a lot within our power to change and to keep doing things that feed this resilience in ourselves."

I find Dr. Emmons' water cooler metaphor a great visual reminder of what can happen when I get really stressed. For instance, when my dream job didn't feed my spirit anymore, it was as though my water cooler had been depleted. I was running out of that precious elixir that kept me happy and healthy. Returning to my love of performing, being kinder at home, taking more time off, even ultimately leaving the dream job all contributed to refilling my water tank.

So what does Dr. Emmons suggest for keeping our water cooler adequately filled and to maximize our resilience? Dr. Emmons tells me that he came up with what he calls "The Seven Roots of Resilience." Naturally, I want to hear all about them!

Dr. Emmons' Seven Roots of Resilience

As we all know, roots are a tree's invisible support: they feed, water, and anchor the tree. Though the roots of resilience can't be seen, like the roots of a tree, they keep us strong, hold us upright, and allow us to withstand life's storms. The first three roots of resilience involve our physical being, the next two consider our mental health, and the final two roots focus on our spirituality.

1. MANAGING YOUR ENERGY

We manage our energy mainly through physical activity. "Exercise is a really good way to keep energy alive," Dr. Emmons says, "because it makes your body respond to a stress that you're purposely giving." What kind of exercise? Studies show that the kind of exercise that will improve mood and boost immunity calls for 30 to 60 minutes a day of aerobic movement, such as swimming, biking, Zumba dancing or fast walking. Why? Because exercise is essentially a stress to the body, and because it stresses the body, the body fights back by releasing a host of chemical reactions that work to improve mood and immunity. (For more on this, see Chapter 4: Establishing a foundation, and the work of *Younger Next Year* authors Crowley and Lodge.)

WHAT IF YOU CAN'T EXERCISE?

Perhaps you are too ill or are without any opportunity to exercise. How can we connect to our physical self? I think of my conversation with Gretchen, the singer and yoga instructor, who put it this way: "Of course there are those moments that are very hard, and you have to search for those things that make you happy." She shifts her weight slightly on the piano bench upon which she is perched. "The things that are very simple, like connecting to your breath and being grateful for your breath, you're never going to lose."

The skeptic in me wonders if it can be this simple. Horrible things happen, and thanking the Creator for my breath will make everything better? But I know from my own experience that just because something is simple doesn't mean it will always be easy. Gretchen is one of the happiest people I know, despite several significant setbacks. She must be on to something. She knows she can bring her mind back to what's most important—namely her breath. The concept is straightforward. But that doesn't make it undemanding; happiness requires more effort than I realized.

2. DIET

Another way to increase resilience has to do with our diet. Food greatly affects our mood because what we eat not only nourishes our bodies but also our brains. For example, high-glucose foods (especially those with a lot of refined sugar and white flour—think donuts, cookies, children's cereals) can trigger roller-coaster mood swings. Lack of protein can make us sluggish and lethargic. "If you're paying attention to eating the foods that are really right for you, it's a really good way to keep brain chemistry at a healthy level," Dr. Emmons instructs. "For some people," he continues, "adding a few nutritional supplements is also good."

3. ALIGNING WITH NATURE (A.K.A. SLEEP AND DAYTIME REST)

The third root is what Dr. Emmons refers to as aligning with nature. "By that I mean recognizing that we are creatures on this planet," adds Dr. Emmons. "We have to pay attention to the rhythm of nature. We have to pay attention to our own body's requirement for rest, especially after we've been really active. From being awake and active during the day and sleeping—sleeping really deeply."

It's no surprise that Americans can use help with our snooze patterns. Many studies show how sleep-deprived we are. Because it is so important to the repair of the body, Dr. Emmons suggests looking to our sleep habits, to try and find ways to "sleep a little bit more perhaps. If one has trouble sleeping, trying to find a good healthy solution to that. Exercise is a good way to promote sleeping well at night. Because again, it's a natural way of tiring out your body."

4. CALMING THE MIND

This is the first of Dr. Emmons' "mental" roots of resilience. The best way to calm the mind is to practice activities that promote mindfulness. I suggest almost any form of sitting or walking meditation. Guided full body relaxation, such as yoga or Qi Gong, can also calm the mind. Formal mindfulness training does wonders for helping us work through challenging emotional states (see Chapter 6: Developing mindfulness). Mindfulness training is essentially being taught how to focus the mind in order to control your attention. In modern life, too often our attention is constantly being pulled in different directions, even though studies* are now proving that multi-tasking is not as effective as we think. Sure you get five things done, but often they are not done well. Perhaps worse, you may have no memory of even doing them, let alone having any pleasure.

Nancy says daily meditation was invaluable in helping her endure the loss of her marriage. Her mind wanted to perseverate on the past or worry about the unknown of what was to come. Daily meditation helps us better tolerate whatever is happening now. It teaches us to accept whatever is coming up in our thoughts, allowing them to pass without getting caught up in them or judging them. When we can do this, even for a few moments, we realize that we are finally being fully alive in the present moment.

MEDITATION VIA REPETITION

Before even getting out of bed, I start each day with a guided meditation. A native Cherokee meditation practice, it includes visualizations and chants that correspond to each of the Chakras. (See www.sunray.org for further information.) This centers me and helps me stay grounded throughout the day. For those who are shy about starting up a meditation practice, consider finding an activity where your mind can truly rest and you can experience being in the moment. Some people achieve a similar state by performing repetitive physical movements, such as crocheting, knitting, woodworking, or sanding. Even walking, running or weight lifting, done in the right way, can bring the mind to a meditative state.

5. PAY ATTENTION TO OUR THOUGHTS AND FEELINGS

To pay attention to our thoughts and feelings, we need to turn toward and not away from them. The goal is to experience all of them, not shun some and embrace others. To recover from a loss, for instance, we actually have to feel it. What got Nancy over her divorce was her ability to turn toward her emotions, as Dr. Emmons suggests. She didn't avoid or deny them. Nor did she try to suppress them with drugs or alcohol, binge eating or shopping. She decided she would welcome them. She found a way to carry them, trusting that, in time, the worst of them would fade. As the saying goes, the more you resist, the more it persists.

For some people, however, looking deeply at their feelings and their self-talk can be terrifying. Hence, they go to great lengths to avoid doing so. When they catch themselves, however, they often can quickly and painlessly counter the downward spiral. For example, a patient of mine who is dealing with recovering from a long illness tends to start getting down on himself whenever he starts to feel tired and weak. We work on countering those thoughts with rational statements, such as, "I am recovering from a major illness. It's normal to need to rest after being ill." Highly anxious people can try to break the hold of their self-talk that starts to awfulize their situations by intentionally countering them with positive affirmations, such as, "Yes, I know the roads are icy. I will drive slowly. I may be late to work, and it will be okay to be late this once. I am okay in this moment."

6. CULTIVATING A GOOD HEART

Dr. Emmons considers the final two roots of resilience "to be in the realm of the spirit or of the heart. And that is cultivating a good heart and creating deep connections." Dr. Emmons also likes to call these roots "learning to love well." One way he helps patients and students open their hearts is through a lovingkindness meditation. This Buddhist meditation focuses on wishing health, prosperity and peace to your immediate family, your friends, acquaintances, and eventually, perhaps even your enemies. By saying loving, kind words to friends as well as enemies, our hearts learn to soften toward those we fear and hate. If your self-esteem is low, it teaches you to feel lovingkindness toward yourself. (See Jack Kornfield's website for his lovingkindess meditation: www.jackkornfield.com).

The goal of open-heartedness is "to develop deep self-acceptance and then compassion for others," Dr. Emmons says, "and then cultivating a real sense of belonging, to a family, a community, a 'tribe,' for example. And finally, attending to deeper relationships to both the inner self as well as to something larger than oneself."

7. CONNECTING DEEPLY WITH OTHERS

There is a wonderful quote by author EM Foster from his novel *Howard's End:* "She would only point out the salvation that was latent in his own soul, and in the soul of every man. Only connect! That was her whole sermon. Only connect the prose and the passion, and both will be exalted, and human love will be seen at its height. Live in fragments no longer. Only connect, and the beast and the monk, robbed of the isolation that is life to either, will die."

Of course we all have a beast and a monk residing inside. The beast strikes out for protection when we feel threatened (the basis of many romantic relationship quarrels, I suspect). The monk represents the part of us that wants to withdraw to avoid being hurt. The phrase "only connect" is often used as shorthand to explain the need to stop denying our need for others in our lives.

Dr. Emmons believes—and I wholeheartedly agree—that loving yourself and investing in healthy, loving relationships is essential to developing true, lasting happiness. This is what Nancy did following her divorce. Despite feeling abandoned and unworthy, she intuitively knew she would do better with support, and she actively sought out the company of others. First she joined a support group with other grieving divorced souls. Later, she made sure to set up times to get together with her family and friends.

As I glance at this list of the Seven Roots of Resiliency, I am stuck by their clarity and power; I've never heard the concept of resilience stated so simply and eloquently. They also remind me of my divorced friend, Nancy. To me, she is the very embodiment of resiliency. As she battled her way back from a devastating loss, she made all seven items a priority. In the end, she created a whole new life that she would not trade for anything in the world.

Resilience is a very close cousin of happiness; the same foundation applies to both. While these seven roots alone are not enough to make us happy, they help make happiness possible. Moreover, in my work with clients and in my own experience, I have discovered that these seven activities also work to help us spring back from difficulty. The same elixir that allows us to be resilient in the face of setbacks also sets the stage for happiness.

THE SEVEN ROOTS OF RESILIENCE, SUMMARIZED

Especially when learning something new, visual reminders can be helpful. I suggest photocopying this summary of the Seven Roots and taping it to your bathroom mirror or another prominent place.

• Manage your energy through engaging in physical activity, eating a diet that is right for you, and getting adequate rest and sleep
• Calm the mind, and pay attention to thoughts and emotions
• Cultivate a good heart, and create deep connections

KEY POINTS

KEY POINTS

• Happier people face the same hardships as everyone
• Fully experiencing their emotions and actively developing resilience allows them to bounce back
• Maintain perspective
• Hold both joy and sorrow
• Manage your energy through moving your body, eating a diet that is right for you, and getting adequate relaxation and sleep
• Calm the mind, and pay attention to your thoughts and emotions
• Cultivate a good heart, and create deep connections

PUTTING IT INTO PRACTICE

ACCEPT that life involves both good times and trying ones. Resist the urge to cling to one or the other. Embrace each fully.

FULLY EXPERIENCE GRIEF Once you've had your sadness over a loss, you can begin to rebuild a life.

MAKE A LIST OF TRAUMAS AND/OR LOSSES

_____

_____

_____

_____

_____

HAVE YOU FULLY GRIEVED? If not, talk it over with a trusted friend or therapist.

APPRECIATE THE HIDDEN GIFTS What did you learn or gain from the loss or trauma? How can you utilize those moving forward?

_____

_____

_____

_____

_____

BE AWARE OF AND GRATEFUL FOR SIMPLE THINGS
See Chapter 5: Expressing thanks, for more suggestions regarding gratitude.

MAKE A LIST OF HOW YOU'VE MANAGED TOUGH TIMES IN THE PAST

_____

_____

_____

_____

_____

_____

Return to the list in times of hardship. It will help remind you of what works for you, and help maintain faith that things will work out.

PRACTICE GOOD SELF-CARE Get physical activity nearly every day. Avoid most junk food. Get adequate relaxation and sleep. Take supplements if needed. For more on this, see Chapter 4: Establishing a foundation.

CALM YOUR MIND Practice relaxation or meditation. Download relaxation and hypnosis apps (many are free) on your smartphone, and listen often. See Chapter 6: Developing mindfulness, for more ideas.

TRAIN THE BRAIN The best way I have found to do this is to take a formal meditation class, such as MBSR (Mindfulness Based Stress Reduction).

SURROUND YOURSELF WITH LOVE Whether wise teachers, mentors, friends or family, spend as much time as possible with people who love you. The unconditional love of pets and other animals also can help tremendously. Love is contagious—if we experience love from others, we believe we are lovable. The reverse, of course, is equally true; if we trust we are lovable, others pick up on that and tend to act accordingly.

BE LOVING TOWARD OTHERS Extending acts of kindness benefits both the giver and recipient. See Chapter 9: Connecting, for more suggestions.

READ Dr. Emmons' books, especially *The Chemistry of Joy* (see Resources FFI).

*Dr. Emmons is an expert in the field of resilience. While he is known mostly for his writing, especially his two books, (*The Chemistry of Joy* and *The Chemistry of Joy Workbook*), he was also one of the first to offer formal instruction on resilience. He developed a ten-week course on resilience that integrates movement, nutrition and supplements, along with the psychology and practice of mindfulness. The goal of the course is to help restore resilience and rediscover joy—even for folks who have been experiencing depression or anxiety for months or years. I took the earliest iteration of the course years ago. It is currently being offered through his collaborative partnership Partners In Resilience www.partnersinresilience.com.

CHAPTER 11

Protecting yourself: News fasts

Everyone knows at least one "news junkie," who can't seem to get enough of the latest information. News junkies read several newspapers each morning, check online news and news blogs frequently throughout the day (workday and weekend), and in the evening switch back and forth between various TV news networks. While they are undoubtedly very well informed, news junkies' up-to-the minute knowledge often comes at the price of social isolation. Relentlessly scanning computer and television screens means not interacting with real people. To add insult to injury, much reported news is "negative" for the simple reason that negative news "sells." While news stories about train accidents or financial ruin easily grab our attention, too many negative stories can dampen our sense of well-being. News junkies love to share stories of doom and gloom, as keeping you well informed makes them feel important. If you want to be happier, however, it may be helpful to avoid over-exposure to negative news.

It was while reading Julia Cameron's book *The Artist's Way* that I first came across the idea of taking news breaks. One of her assignments to increase creativity is to take a week of what she calls "reading deprivation." She believes, "For most blocked creatives, reading is an addiction. We gobble the words of others rather than digest our own thoughts and feelings, rather than cook up something of our own." Much as I love to read, I like to think of reading vacations (and news fasts) as cleansing the palate in between courses of a fine, multiple-course meal. Despite loads of resistance (I nearly always read a chapter or two of an engrossing novel before bed, and I can't seem to pass a newsstand without perusing the headlines), I tried it a few years ago. Even after just a few days without the news or other reading, my senses were sharper and my emotions more accessible. I found I was much more in touch with the present moment.

While I was never a news junkie myself, I've certainly experimented with extremes in this arena. For years, the only station I played while driving was Minnesota Public Radio. It didn't take long for me to feel as though the announcers were my friends, their familiar voices soothing and informing me as I drove. I'd arrive at my destination stewing over the stupidity of some random senator's remarks and then spend time at my appointment complaining.

After a news fast, despite my fondness for the MPR announcers, I find I'm far happier singing along to the FM radio or songs on my iPhone on my way to and from work, errands, and appointments. I tend to reach journey's end in a good mood. I daresay I'm more creative as well. I've now gone years with only occasional and brief forays into MPR.

Cameron was ahead of her time, as scientists have confirmed the wisdom of news fasts. In their book, *Abundance*, Peter H. Diamandis and Steven Kotler write, "A quick glance at the headlines is enough to set anybody on edge and—with the endless media stream that has lately become our lives—it's hard to get away from those headlines. Worse, evolution shaped the human brain to be acutely aware of all potential dangers....this dire combination has a profound impact on human perception: It literally shuts off our ability to take in good news." Whoa. Our inborn wiring combined with our 24/7 news cycle—which naturally tends to emphasize bad news—leads to an inability to see the good. Now that's a scary headline.

"I quit watching television," Jenn tells me during her interview, nodding her head slightly. "I haven't had cable or watched television in three years. And I don't pay attention to the news. I just deal with what's right here," she says. Arms wide and hands open, her nonverbals indicate the world that's right in front of her. Doing so doesn't automatically come guilt-free, however. "I feel irresponsible when it comes to that," Jenn says, a hint of self-reproach in her tone, "because I feel like I should know what's going on in the world. But at the same time, that was driving me insane. It was this negative, so I just had to let it go."

How does she handle the need to know important events? She came up with a solution and provides the following example: "When it comes to elections, I do my research online," Jenn says. "The TV ads are negative anyway, and they're so horrible. So I do my own research. So I don't feel irresponsible in that way. Sometimes I feel like I should know what's going on with our military and all of that, but I can't do anything about it. So I have to start here." As before, Jenn motions toward the space between us.

When I ask Mia at her interview how she handles the negativity of media news, she explains, "Happiness for me has something to do with letting things be okay the way that they are," she says. "Because they're okay."

Wait a minute, I think. Not everything is "okay." A lot of horrible things happen every day. I ask Mia to explain how bad news can be "okay." Mia shoots me a disapproving look, as though I should know better, but then she pauses and takes a breath. "I think it's a both/and," she tells me. "I think there are really terrible things that happen in the world, and I think there is some way in which—because I've cultivated this sense of contentedness and happiness—I can send that wish out to that terrible situation. So I don't necessarily separate myself from it."

I love this idea that noticing when there is suffering in the world, Mia sends a silent blessing to those in need. In any situation, she can at least do that. And, in saying she doesn't separate herself from the suffering, she emphasizes how we are all interconnected, regardless of our circumstances. Mia pauses to add, "I don't do a lot of media, because I find that there is so much bad news, and if I put my attention there, I feel it differently. So, I'm not really 'Captain Current Events.'" (I can't help but grin at the image of a caped news crusader.)

A lot of people, I bet, can relate. Who hasn't wondered if they'd be better off not focusing on horrors thousands of miles away?

But isn't avoiding the news sticking our heads in the sand? "Do you think you are in denial about this?" I ask. "Maybe," Mia replies, looking thoughtful. "I feel like I have a sense about what goes on in the world, and I also think I really have this reference point of basic goodness. Even with terrible conflict, people hurting each other, etcetera, there's a place in me that believes at some level this is a situation that is trying to find more health."

This sounds to me similar to the symptoms we get when we're sick—the runny nose, fatigue, and fever—that are actually the body's attempt to return to health. "Ah, I see. You're not denying the existence of terrible news," I say to Mia. "You're saying there's still goodness in it."

"Yes. I'm saying that," Mia says, sounding satisfied.

Dr. Emmons, having overheard the exchange, comments later. "Mia talked about choosing not to listen to the media, for example, and I think you asked a question, 'Is that denial?'"

Yes, that was the question. Naturally I'm curious to hear his take. "Well, in a way, yes," Dr. Emmons acknowledges, his brow furrowing, but he quickly adds, "In another way, it's a very conscious choice to be attentive about what she's feeding herself, and what she's putting into her mind, because, in this case, it affects how she feels. And so, the same things are happening out there in the world for her as to others, but she's choosing to keep her focus on things in a more positive way. That's just being conscious about it. That's not denial in my book," Dr. Emmons maintains, "because she's making a very conscious choice. She's doing it on purpose."

Here, Dr. Emmons is carefully discerning. He's pointing out the importance of acknowledging the truth that suffering exists, as Mia does. She doesn't pretend everyone is happy. She is aware of her own content-edness, and from that place of equanimity and stability sends comforting wishes and goodwill to those in need. She accepts that there is imperfection in the world and does what she can, even if it is something as simple as offering a prayer.

I think that Dr. Emmons is also drawing a comparison: what we expose to our minds is similar to choosing what foods we eat. Notice the words he selects: "a conscious choice to be attentive about what she's feeding herself." He's a big promoter of how nutritional choices affect our moods. When athletes choose not to consume large quantities of refined sugar, for instance, we don't accuse them of denying that sugar exists. They simply decide not to ingest it to help them achieve a particular goal.

Nutritionists like to say that there's nothing wrong with the occasional favorite junk food. Why not apply that concept to the news? Get just enough so we're informed and satisfied, and so we aren't ignorant and don't feel deprived. Balance, of course, is key. Too much news and we are sent over the edge into negativity.

"There just are all kinds of distractions," mentions Dr. Emmons. "Many of them are things that we choose. How we spend our free time. All kinds of electronic things. They're very, very interesting, but they also have a tendency to put our minds in a little bit more of a distracted state. So I think there is such a huge need today, more so than ever perhaps, for us to intentionally decide that we are going to cultivate greater presence and awareness. Otherwise, it won't happen automatically." In other words, reducing our exposure to electronic distractions can help us be more mindful.

Don't get me wrong, I'm not a teetotaler. When I run on the treadmill, I love flipping back and forth between various morning news shows. On Sundays, I relish sleeping in and then leisurely perusing the *Minneapolis Star Tribune*, or, on a really good day, *The New York Times*. I love to feel the paper crinkling in my hands as I turn the pages.

Most days, I turn to the Internet for my daily dose of the goings on in the world. I scan the headlines and click on the stories I want to know more about. I subscribe to email alerts of causes I care deeply about and sign several electronic petitions every day. I send letters to my elected officials expressing my views. I donate money to causes I believe in. I pick up litter. I vote. I care deeply about the suffering of others. Like Mia, I send silent blessings their way. When I want or need to watch upsetting news stories, I try to do so with a friend or family member. Company seems to help soften the blow.

Would reducing our exposure to the news increase our happiness? It just might be worth a try.

KEY POINTS

KEY POINTS

- Most of the people I interviewed in my happiness videos avoid news overexposure
- Instead, focus on positive events and what you can influence
- Don't, however, deny suffering
- Find a way to be aware of suffering and remain happy
- Because our brains are wired to focus on negative news and the news cycle is now 24/7, our ability to resist becoming negative is being severely tested
- Consider being more deliberate about when and how you "consume" news, much as you might be deliberate about your nutritional choices

PUTTING IT INTO PRACTICE

INVENTORY Check the headlines of the nearest newspaper. Compare how many "positive" news stories you find to every negative one

_____

_____

_____

_____

_____

_____

LIMIT your exposure to the news. Slowly decrease it over time, replacing it with other activities you enjoy.

PRACTICE MODERATION Like foods, consume media within sensible limits.

REDUCE USE OF ELECTRONICS Think "high touch over high tech." Stop by a coworker's cube instead of sending that email. Meet a friend for coffee or a game of golf. Call your friend instead of text or PM.

EXPERIMENT WITH NEWS FASTS Wean yourself slowly. But consider spending half a day, then a whole day, then a weekend, etc., slowly increasing the time away from the headlines. Record how you feel.

NEWS MEDIA DAY

Upon Awakening
Mood
BAD 1 2 3 4 5 6 7 GREAT
Clarity of Thought
CLOUDY 1 2 3 4 5 6 7 CLEAR

An hour after breakfast
Mood
BAD 1 2 3 4 5 6 7 GREAT
Clarity of Thought
CLOUDY 1 2 3 4 5 6 7 CLEAR

Mid-afternoon
Mood
BAD 1 2 3 4 5 6 7 GREAT
Clarity of Thought
CLOUDY 1 2 3 4 5 6 7 CLEAR

NEWS FAST DAY

Upon Awakening
Mood
BAD 1 2 3 4 5 6 7 GREAT
Clarity of Thought
CLOUDY 1 2 3 4 5 6 7 CLEAR

An hour after breakfast
Mood
BAD 1 2 3 4 5 6 7 GREAT
Clarity of Thought
CLOUDY 1 2 3 4 5 6 7 CLEAR

Mid-afternoon
Mood
BAD 1 2 3 4 5 6 7 GREAT
Clarity of Thought
CLOUDY 1 2 3 4 5 6 7 CLEAR

Mid-evening
Mood
BAD 1 2 3 4 5 6 7 GREAT
Clarity of Thought
CLOUDY 1 2 3 4 5 6 7 CLEAR

Mid-evening
Mood
BAD 1 2 3 4 5 6 7 GREAT
Clarity of Thought
CLOUDY 1 2 3 4 5 6 7 CLEAR

Bedtime
Mood
BAD 1 2 3 4 5 6 7 GREAT
Clarity of Thought
CLOUDY 1 2 3 4 5 6 7 CLEAR

Bedtime
Mood
BAD 1 2 3 4 5 6 7 GREAT
Clarity of Thought
CLOUDY 1 2 3 4 5 6 7 CLEAR

SWITCH THE SOURCE Obtain news from sources you have more control of, such as the Internet or the paper instead of television.

IDENTIFY ACTION STEPS Take today's headlines. Identify what is in your control regarding it. For example, can you donate money? Can you volunteer? Write a letter to the editor? Contact your elected officials?

TODAY'S HEADLINES	WHAT I CAN DO	CHECK WHEN COMPLETE
_____	_____	_____
_____	_____	_____
_____	_____	_____
_____	_____	_____
_____	_____	_____
_____	_____	_____

SEND BLESSINGS Knowing others suffer, send positive blessings their way. Wish them relief. Imagine them free of their suffering.

ACT LOCALLY Identify the causes that most concern you: education, economic development, the environment, human rights, etc. What can you do about them within your own household? Your neighborhood? Your workplace? Your faith community? Your city or town?

_____

_____

_____

_____

_____

Make a list of all the good things that happened today, whether in the media or not (most of it likely isn't)

_____

_____

_____

_____

_____

CONSUME IN COMPANY When you do choose to watch the news, do so with a friend or family member. Talk about what you've seen, how it makes you feel, and what you can do about it.

CHAPTER 12

Giving back without depleting: Gifts from the heart

Deep in the Green Mountains of Vermont, I sit in a tiny, rickety lawn chair inside a small, grey, clapboard structure often called "the meeting-house." Located on a gorgeous piece of property formally known as the Peace Village, most of us present, sitting shoulder to shoulder, simply refer to it as "The Land." Sunray Meditation Society offers meditation and sacred Native American ceremonies and teachings year round.

Once every summer, an annual gathering of devoted, advanced students from around the world descends to commune, work, and learn. Think of it as an international conference where most of us camp and many of the activities are held outdoors. I listen intently as Venerable Dhyani Ywahoo, a Cherokee who is the founder of Sunray Meditation Society, talks about the status of the organization. Sunray offers Native American healing teachings and rituals that promote personal and planetary peace. I have been studying with Venerable Dhyani for five years; she is instrumental in helping me learn to meditate and be kinder to others, the earth, and myself.

Suddenly, Venerable Dhyani stops her talk and looks deeply at the students in the room—some from as far away as Germany. She has been urging us to become more active in helping. "When you see a need," she implores, "do it."

I take her words to heart, but soon find myself fretting about all the needs I see in the world. There are so many, it's overwhelming—how can one person make a dent in issues as monumental as hunger, pollution, poverty, and illiteracy? The list seems endless. If I try to take care of every one of those needs by myself, I'll never have time for my job or my family, let alone sleep or meditation. And yet, clearly I am being instructed to help. Feeling overwhelmed, I decide to ask Venerable Dhyani about this dilemma. She is such a presence; even when she is addressing a crowd, I always feel that she is talking just to me. This time, her kind, green eyes indeed focus on me, soothing the slight trepidation and embarrassment I feel at asking her a question. (I'm always slightly star-struck in her presence). She takes a breath. In her lyrical, reassuring voice she says, "Then you do what you can." This simple statement cuts through my confusion; I no longer feel the weight of the world on my shoulders—I can do as much as I am able.

How I wish I had heard those wise words before 1996, when I learned of the first Twin Cities to Chicago AIDS bikeathon. This 500 mile ride was to be completed in six days. Organizers wanted 1,500 riders to raise $1,200 each, with the proceeds to be distributed between 12 AIDS charities. At the time, that struck me as a huge sum of money, but I was game to try. Having been an avid biker for years, I had long dreamed of completing a multi-state bike ride, but I could never figure out the logistics. Here, all that was taken care of. The route was laid out, various towns along the way hosted large campsites, the organizers would provide all meals, and our luggage would be transported for us. We could even take a hot shower each night. After fundraising, "all" we had to do was ride 60 to 100 miles a day and pitch a tent each night.

Part of the pull was that I believed I should do something to help with the AIDS crisis. There are many causes I care about, but as a gay man, this one hit particularly close to home. I had friends, clients, and coworkers with HIV or AIDS. It didn't escape me that AIDS fundraising events tend to have fewer attendees and so fewer contributors.

I went to one brief informational meeting and signed up. In retrospect,

I realize I chose to overlook the serious misgivings I was having. My biggest hesitation? Each rider was required to raise the $1,200 minimum on their own, and I hated asking people for money. Plus, I had only six months to get my body in shape to survive the 500-mile bike ride. The most I had ever biked in one day was maybe 40 miles at best; I would have to work up to at least twice that to keep up and finish in six days. Training like that would take much of my free time for the next half year.

The part of me that believed I had to do something substantial about an issue I cared about caused me to suppress another inner voice, which was telling me to take a few days to think about this.

Anxiety over potentially failing to raise the required money catapulted me into overdrive. I disregarded my shyness about asking people for money and went all out. I asked everyone I could think of for donations: I sent out direct mail requests and hosted fundraising parties. I even mentioned it to strangers on the street. In the end, I managed to raise 10 times the minimum.

Meanwhile, I started training like a fiend, biking for hours up and down the hills and through the prairies of east-central Minnesota. Straddled on my beat-up red Trek 7500, I rode at least 25 miles each day during the week. On Saturdays and Sundays, I doubled or tripled that. It was hard going. I started to miss my weekends at home with Greg, and I missed my friends. I hadn't seen a movie in what felt like ages.

Then, I had an epiphany. I was on a training ride one hot, muggy summer afternoon. Near the top of a desolate hill somewhere far west of Minneapolis, I simply stopped in my tracks and reached for my familiar plastic bottle. Squeezing out a sip of tepid water and wiping my brow with the meshed back of my smelly black riding glove, it hit me. I was lonely. I was tired. I wasn't enjoying myself. I didn't want to do this any more.

On one level these feelings surprised me, but it also felt good to finally let them arise after I had been forcing them down for so long. While I liked biking a lot—as a hobby—this effort required turning it into a second job. Plus, my true strengths and talents lay elsewhere. I would much rather have done something that reflected more of my heart, say acting in a performance that raised money for AIDS or raising awareness through teaching.

It was too late, however, to back out. Hundreds of kind people had donated money for each mile I rode, and their checks were cashed. What was I going to do? Pay them back out of my own pocket? I had made a commitment, and I had already put so much into it. Sharing my doubts with no one, I rode on. The weight on my shoulders felt crushing.

Though my heart was not fully in it, I completed the Ride—all 500 miles, from the Minneapolis Convention Center to Chicago's Lincoln Park—in six days. Parts of the Ride were grueling. July humidity in the Midwest can be brutal. (That's when I learned electrolyte drinks really do work!) Some of the Wisconsin hills were pure evil. Downshifting to low gear on one monster hill, I passed other riders who had long since dismounted to walk their bikes up the steep incline. But they encouraged me on. "Keep going . . . you can do it . . . you're special," they unselfishly cheered. I beam now at the memory, as I did at the time.

In many ways, the AIDS Ride was a good experience. My brother Joe drove from Michigan and also rode, so I wasn't alone. Many of the other riders I met along the way were amazing, each with a profound, inspiring story. (I remain in touch with several of them to this day). I got in great shape. As punishing as the Ride was, I did it, and I felt proud of myself. But for all that, as an accomplishment, the Ride felt a bit hollow. It wasn't until I experienced other accomplishments undertaken for the right reasons that I realized the problem. I did the AIDS Ride because I felt guilty for the blessings I had in my life, while so many others were suffering. It wasn't until I volunteered for other activities with a full, glad, open heart that I noticed the difference.

I learned the hard way that guilt is not the best motivation for taking action. That much fundraising and biking required far too much time and energy. In the end, I felt depleted. I got caught up in my co-dependent belief that if I can do something, I *should* do it. Had I truly wanted to complete the Ride, the herculean effort would have been worthwhile. But without my full, true, open heart, I experienced little joy. Why? I am not a hardcore biker. Just because you enjoy something doesn't mean you will continue to like it if you have to do a whole lot of it. I realized then that it is important not to overdo an activity, especially in relation to giving. Our time and energy are not infinite; we need to protect these assets. With the Ride, I felt I had given 98% with a 2% return.

I am not saying the AIDS Ride stopped me from supporting and giving to HIV/AIDS organizations. It didn't. But it did harm my love of cycling. Before the Ride, I regularly rode around town or on picturesque trails for hours, for the sheer fun of it. I felt so free on my bike. While I now occasionally get out my bike, I'm not the cycling aficionado I once was. It's as though once I associated biking with obligation, I never fully recovered. I miss the passion I felt, if not long-distance riding itself. Who knows, it may yet return.

THE SIX-MONTH RESENTMENT QUESTION

One of my interviewees, Barry, the Connecticut counseling center director, had a similar insight about volunteering. "I used to say 'yes' to everything. Oh my god, it was such a nightmare," Barry says. "Now I only say yes to things I at least want to do. So I don't feel resentful, I ask myself, 'In six months will I be resentful that I agreed to do this?' If the answer is yes, I won't do it." For Barry, there needs to be an alignment between doing things well and doing things he loves. That alignment fuels his wellbeing and happiness.

Another fallout of the AIDS Ride was that I didn't volunteer for anything for quite a while. Emotionally and physically exhausted, I felt I had given more than enough blood to a good cause. The message is clear: be careful what you say "Yes" to. Unforeseen consequences may ensue.

There certainly is a silver lining to this story. My AIDS Ride experience taught me the importance of doing things with my whole heart—to take on jobs I have real passion for. With my soul thus electrified, I am involved in events and create objects that are infused with the joy with which I offer them. Plus, when I do things I love, I'm happier, which undoubtedly affects those around me. When I give from the heart, there is more return on the investment; my energy isn't as depleted. Even if I feel fatigue at times from the effort, ultimately my energy actually increases. That's what happens when we follow our bliss.

For causes I have less interest in (or the skills for), I recall Venerable Dhyani. I see her in that crowded room in the Peace Village outside of Bristol, Vermont, perched on the edge of her chair, with her impeccable posture. "Do what you can." For me, that means doing exactly that, what I can. Sometimes that is signing a petition, and others times it means writing a check or even taking a page from Mia's book and saying a prayer.

When we are contemplating volunteering, it is vital to consider our emotions and our resources. We need to tune in to all our feelings, especially negative ones like guilt. We experience guilt when we say "no" to something we "should" do, and we feel resentment when we say "yes" to something we don't want to do. As you ponder what is behind your decisions, allow yourself to experience these feelings if they are arising. If we thwart the full spectrum of our emotions—the pleasant as well as the unpleasant ones—we can't tune in to what is really going on in the gut, the heart, and the soul.

Now when I'm asked to do things, I try to turn my attention inward and search my heart and soul. Before agreeing, I ask myself: Does my body tell me this is something I really want to do? How fun does it sound? Like Barry, I ask if in six months I will feel resentful if I say yes. When I answer these questions truthfully, my answer is certain to align with my heart.

Once I became a parent, I discovered that volunteering at my son's school did align with my heart. It made me feel happy and fulfilled. These were short-term but meaningful commitments that allowed me to help my son's teachers and classmates and made me feel part of the school community. I got back as much as I put in.

Just think. If we all acted from our hearts and did things that bring us joy, wouldn't there be fewer causes to address?

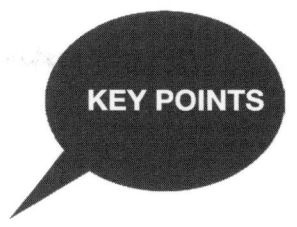

KEY POINTS

KEY POINTS

- Do what you can
- Do what you love
- Trust your intuition
- Listen to your heart
- It's okay to wait a few days before making a decision
- It's okay to say no
- Remember, "No" is a complete sentence. You don't need to justify why you are saying it

PUTTING IT INTO PRACTICE

BEWARE OF "SHOULDS" Whenever you catch yourself using the dreaded "should" word, as in "I should volunteer," ask yourself what you want to do in your heart. If you're not used to doing so, it may take some time for your intuition to "wake up." Maybe "sleep" will come to mind. This may indeed be a sign that you need some rest. Get the rest, and then see what you can contribute.

CAUSES I'M PASSIONATE ABOUT   WHAT I'D LIKE TO DO ABOUT THEM

_____   _____

_____   _____

_____   _____

_____   _____

_____   _____

ACCEPT volunteer tasks when your heart is drawn to them and when you know you can complete them without resentment.

CONTRIBUTE IN OTHER WAYS For causes you care about but don't have the skills or interest in working directly on, you can offer to provide meals or help with child care for other volunteers. Or consider donating money.

WRITE LETTERS TO THE EDITOR regarding causes that are important to you. They actually do make a difference.

SIGN PETITIONS Elected officials and retailers like to keep people happy. Collective action does sway policy and decisions.

LET YOUR FEET DO THE TALKING Don't shop at businesses whose practices fail to reflect your values.

VOTE. Enough said.

DISCERN AND USE GUILT Feelings of guilt can help guide us in the right direction, but we must dig deeply into the cause of the feelings. If it's "pure" guilt, you've acted in violation of your values. A repair or apology is warranted, and you need to change your ways. Often, however, we feel guilty when we needn't. If you haven't erred, you don't need to feel guilt. Let go of this kind of unproductive shame.

DO WHAT YOU CAN/DO AS MUCH AS YOU CAN Being an activist is a great thing. If you burn yourself out, however, you can't do well for anyone. Do as much you can. Then rest.

CHAPTER 13

Believing in yourself: Countertop wisdom

My interviewee Barry is one of the happiest people I have ever encountered. We met at a national conference for counseling center directors. Like a magnet, people are drawn to his positive energy, kindness, and goodwill. When I interview him in his Connecticut home, I am struck by his positive attitude. "Not only do I consider the glass half full," he tells me, "I'm pleased just to have the glass!"

While many of us must work at being happy, it seems to come naturally to Barry. Like the other people I interviewed, Barry realizes that happiness is actually a constellation of certain key attitudes and beliefs that allow him to stay true to his values.

But I wanted to know what happens when someone with a good attitude is confronted with bad news, an accident, or a malicious act?

Remaining Happy in the Face of Trouble

Barry's test came several years ago while he was working as a counselor at a large, southern university. When his partner, Tom, suddenly became ill, Barry missed a day of work to take him to the doctor. Returning to work the next day—following university policy he had learned at employee orientation—Barry submitted for a day of family sick leave.

Evidently this policy was not going to apply in Barry's case. "You need to take it as a vacation day," the HR department instructed in its reply, rejecting his claim out of hand.

Puzzled, Barry asked for an explanation. "Your relationship is not recognized," he was told. "He's not your husband. You don't have a wife. He's not your kid. It doesn't fit the university's definition of family."

"I was like, are you fricking kidding me?" Barry says, his voice incredulous. He appealed the HR ruling, but the appeal was promptly denied.

Barry did not give up. "I always had the idea, in that kind of situation, if someone said 'No' to me, you were just the wrong person to be talking to. 'No' never meant no. No meant, 'I will find someone else to talk to,'" Barry says, with a characteristic shrug. When you don't take things personally, you are able to be resilient; instead of breaking, you can bend. (For more on resilience, see Chapter 10: Bouncing back with resilience.)

Obstacles often deter less happy people who tend to assume that any barrier is intended just for them, presented purposely and uniquely to get in their way. For example, when they aren't hired for a job, they believe it is a reflection of their intrinsic worth. Or, when a contractor doesn't return a call, less happy people might be inclined to procrastinate or even give up on repairing the roof. Then, when the next rainstorm hits, they're more discouraged than ever, using it as evidence of what to them is an obvious truth: "Bad things always happen to me." Happier people, in contrast, aren't so easily discouraged. Upon not getting a particular job, they might shrug and say something like, "Maybe they found someone with more experience. There must be something better for me out there." When a contractor doesn't return a call, happier folks are more likely to promptly follow up with an email or find a different professional for the job.

Barry kept marching up the bureaucratic ladder. In a display of great tenacity and clear conviction, he kept filing appeal after appeal. Although the battle went on for months, he remained resolute. "It was unreasonable for me to do the same work as everyone else and get different benefits," Barry explains, a solemn expression darkening his usually amiable features.

Barry began receiving seemingly endless correspondence from university officials. One letter is particularly memorable. Says Barry: "I got one that was basically a cease and desist letter, in effect saying your job is in jeopardy if you continue to be insubordinate. I was furious. I'm going to get the fricking ACLU in here. You'll get press that you won't want. Whether it's successful or not, I will make sure you get press you don't want."

Being angry at a setback or obstacle is normal. Many people, however, see anger in a negative light. They associate anger with being abusive. But in reality, anger is a healthy response to an upsetting situation. To me, anger is often an indication from our insides that there is something that we need to do to protect, defend, or take care of. As a mentor once told me, "Anger is the emotion of determination."

We can use anger to energize us to take action. But if we suppress anger, we risk falling into a trap of passivity, and therefore fail to take needed action. Such passivity essentially encourages—and teaches—others to take advantage of us. This is a shorthand definition of learned helplessness.

Barry used his anger at the policy's injustice to fuel his resolve to fight it. He was careful, however, not to become obsessed or consumed. How do you keep from letting a battle for justice overtake you?

First you need to be aware that you might be getting obsessed. This is where mindfulness practices can be really helpful. Mindfulness helps us wake up to what is happening and make a choice to change our focus. (See Chapter 6: Developing mindfulness.) Second, doing something physical is a great antidote to obsessive thinking. Getting into the body helps counter all that mental rumination. Third, talking about it with a trusted friend or therapist can be invaluable. Venting can dispel troubling emotions and clarify thoughts and intentions.

Sharing the burden with others was another important piece in Barry's battle. He realized the injustice wasn't just about him. It affected others, as well. As he tells me, "Well, is this all about me? That's not a good thing. I'm going to start rallying staff and faculty together."

A natural organizer, Barry formed a gay and lesbian staff and faculty group to add strength to his appeals. In time, he also found that this new community went far beyond his particular HR issue. New friendships were formed among various members. When other injustices were encountered, the group was in place to lend assistance. As anyone who has been involved in groups knows, a well-functioning group is there in times of great need, as well as during the inevitable challenges of everyday life.

Fueled both by his own commitment and that of his support community, Barry just kept writing appeals. Eventually, the matter landed on the desk of the university president, who apparently thought the ruling was just as ridiculous as Barry did. "When the president got it, he said, 'Let's change this!'" Barry's whole face lights up as he recalls the sweet taste of victory. "It was awesome."

I hear pride in Barry's voice. "I never give up," he says. I ask him where he thinks his persistence comes from. Barry tells me about going to religious school as a boy. "I acquired my sense of social justice from my teachers," he says, his voice suddenly deeper. "They all had little tattoos on their arms." Forcibly applied by Nazis, these dehumanizing tattoos were identification numbers. Many of Barry's teachers, you see, were Holocaust survivors.

From his teachers' experiences, Barry learned how discipline, focus, finding like-minded comrades, and perseverance play a key role in helping overcome self-doubt.

"I think it's an assertive person's world," Barry tells me. "That's an operating philosophy. I try not to wait. Waiting sort of leaves me waiting. So if I think, 'Oh, we should go do that. Oh, that would be cool if that happened for us.' I think, well, what are we going to do about it? We have to go do something about it; otherwise it's not going to happen. It's not an aggressive person's world. But I do think it's an assertive person's world."

Happier people believe that their efforts matter and make a difference. They trust that they can advocate for themselves. They have what is called "agency," meaning the capacity to make independent choices.

Not infrequently, the people who come to see me for life-coaching or therapy have great difficulty taking action on their own behalf. They are trapped in a pattern of passivity and learned helplessness. These people often have repeated, vivid memories of experiences where they attempted to stand up for themselves, but were ignored, mocked, or even punished for it. Thus, they came to believe that nothing they do will make any difference.

BEWARE THE FALSE 'I DON'T KNOW'

Not infrequently, I hear lonely clients claim, "I don't know how to meet people." When I ask how they met friends before, they say things like "we met in school," "we were roommates," "we were on the same team." Great, I say, and then I keep gently pressing. What happened at school or on the team? How did you start talking, specifically? Most of them say that they talked about common interests. The same elements apply today, I tell them. The best way to meet people is to find those who share your interests. I urge my clients to take a class in an area they have real interest, perhaps a how-to class or even a seminar for their job. Or join a choir or a tennis league. It can be anything, just so long as they are in a group where everyone is doing the same thing. Too often "I don't know how to meet people" really means, "I'm scared." Another way to break through such blocks is to assume you do know what to do. Ask, What would you do if you did know how to meet people?

An overabundance of such painful experiences can result in an "emotional paralysis," where people believe they are incapable of making any lasting change. They come to see themselves as victims of outside circumstances, even though their circumstances may have changed. For example, say a child playing on a girl's soccer team is repeatedly ridiculed for her lack of athletic ability by one of the team's stars. Even as an adult, she may refuse to do anything remotely athletic. Sometimes the wounding goes so deep that this kind of belief becomes generalized, causing people to take no risks in any area. This becomes a self-fulfilling prophecy, of course. They believe they can't do anything, and that becomes true—not because they can't, but because they don't. As some of my clients have told me, such beliefs "give me permission not to try."

Countertop Wisdom: "I Think I Can"

My brother-in-law Brian provides a potent counterpoint to learned helplessness. Having known him for years (I even lived with him one summer), I know Brian is highly social and loves to laugh, never passing an opportunity to crack a joke. He's also a very hard worker and has a strong sense of himself. Brian's optimism and belief in himself allow him to succeed and excel. But how exactly does that happen? As I ponder the question, I flash back to the transformation of his and my eldest sister Mary Beth's kitchen in their first home. This was in the late 1980s, and, newly married, Mary Beth and Brian were living in a charming area. The tree-lined streets led to one-and-a-half story brick houses that were built in the 1930s to accommodate the burgeoning number of Detroit autoworkers. Like Mary Beth and Brian, lots of young families were starting their lives in this idyllic neighborhood.

The stately houses were aging, however, and seriously needed upgrades. When I visited shortly after they moved in, the kitchen was torn up, with stuff all over the place. Brian was in the midst of renovating it. My jaw dropped, because I knew Brian had zero experience doing any kind of renovating work. But there he was with a Number 2 pencil tucked behind his ear and a tape measure in hand.

I can still see him in that kitchen measuring the old yellow Formica countertop and scribbling notes on a small white pad. With no prior experience or special training, Brian explains that he is going to rip out the old Formica all by himself and put in a new countertop that he cut himself. More than impressed, I am stunned. How could he just assume he can do that?

I could never do that, I thought. How can Brian? As I stood there, my mouth forming an "O" in awe, it came to me in a flash. He was able to do so because he believed he could. Yes, I know it sounds trite, but it's true nonetheless. Not only did he imagine himself doing it (visualization), he trusted he could do it (belief).

It's through imagination and trust that happier people make things happen. I think of my clean-cut Minnesotan interviewee Ryan who gets excited as he shares his take on this make-it-happen concept. "It's like that movie *The Matrix*," he tells me. "He believes he can fly, he can do it. But the moment he believes he can't, he won't. That's our life. I believe we can do anything. The only thing that's holding us back right now is ourselves, because we don't fully believe." As Ryan pauses for a moment, I wonder if he is thinking about his own experience of setting his mind to become a filmmaker before he even knew what filmmakers did. He adds, "When you think about extraordinary individuals throughout history and the things they were able to create and the things they were able to do, they believed in themselves," he says. His volume rises in excitement. "They didn't see those limitations. They thought, 'I could do anything.'" Ryan has a point. He went from being a near-college-dropout to a filmmaker in part because he believed he could.

It's the same with Brian, my brother-in-law, and his kitchen. First, he believed he could do it. Then he broke it down into manageable steps. While he undoubtedly made mistakes, he didn't let that discourage him; he worked them out. I suspect he did not take any setbacks personally. If he made a mistake, he simply took it in stride and tried again. He trusted himself to find the right answer. His enthusiasm helped keep him going beyond the inevitable setbacks of sailing in unchartered territory.

We all know unhappy people who stay stuck because they don't believe in themselves. They fail to try new things—and criticize others who do. Happy people, in contrast, think differently. They do try new things. And if they fail, they are not surprised, because it is something new they are doing.

By utilizing all our resources—including courage, community, creativity, and especially persistence and belief in ourselves—we make things happen. And sometimes, even greater things come from staying with it, such as a new kitchen counter, or a faculty and staff LGBT organization.

KEY POINTS

- If you truly believe you can do it, you probably can
- Persistence often pays off
- Fighting righteous causes can lead to community
- Happier people take setbacks less personally
- Setbacks often lead to unexpected—and even greater—results than anticipated
- "It's an assertive person's world"
- Positive role models help us overcome self-doubt

PUTTING IT INTO PRACTICE

OVERCOMING RESISTANCE

I met Pam in a community theater production. A stay-at-home mom, she was in her late 40s with two children and a loving husband. With her girls in their early teens, she was beginning to feel restless and less fulfilled than when the girls were younger and "needed her more." She had a dream she always wanted to fulfill.

1. Pam wanted to be in a musical but never tried out for one.
2. She wasn't sure she could do it; she'd always wanted to, but she had no formal experience acting or dancing. Moreover, she was afraid it would take her away from time with her growing kids.
3. She found a community theater that welcomed families. She and her daughters tried out for a local musical production and got parts in the chorus.

LIST three things you've always wanted to do but haven't:

(example: I always wanted to tap dance.*)

1. _____

2. _____

3. _____

*NOTE: Here we must consider certain fundamental limits. In my case, for example, standing 5'6" and weighing 160, I'm unlikely to become a linebacker in the NFL. If football is my thing, it may be wise for me to explore other ways of engaging my passion.

WRITE what's kept you from doing them:

(example: I had no time to learn it.)

1. _____

2. _____

3. _____

4. _____

5. _____

IDENTIFY what you can do to make those there things happen. If you're having trouble, look at the ideas below, and come back to complete this section:

(example: I found time by cutting down on TV watching.)

1. _____

2. _____

3. _____

4. _____

5. _____

VISUALIZE SUCCESS

Make a "mental movie." See yourself taking the steps necessary to achieve your goal. Imagine yourself facing setbacks with equanimity. Engage all your senses. What will you see, touch, smell, taste, and hear when you've accomplished your goal—and along the way?

TAKE IT PUBLIC
Announcing your intentions to make a change increases the likelihood that you will persevere.

ASK FOR WHAT YOU NEED
Recruit trusted comrades to help you achieve your goal. Be specific about what you'd like them to do. Do you need a cheerleader? Assign someone that role. A mentor or coach? Find one. Someone to listen when doubts come up? Ask a friend to be on "stand by," a quick phone call away.

TAKE NOTHING PERSONALLY
It can be tempting to interpret setbacks as a message from beyond that you're not meant to do it. It may be the universe's way of telling you there are unexpected lessons along the way. Take from each experience what you can. It's fine to reassess along the way; your goal may change. But if it's truly in your heart, keep finding ways to do what you love.

BE CREATIVE
When roadblocks and setbacks appear, see if there is another way.

EXERCISE DISCIPLINE
Achieving goals takes more than visualizing, of course. Action is required, and often similar actions need to be repeated over and over again. So whether it's practicing the piano or getting a promotion, put in time and effort. This book would not have been completed, for instance, had I not set large chunks of time in my calendar or if I allowed distractions to keep me from writing.

TAKE BREAKS
On the other hand, don't be so persistent that you burn yourself out by not getting the rest you need. All creative endeavors and learning require adequate "down time" to percolate. During the writing of this book, I took several extended breaks—some as long as a year. When I

tried to force the writing, I didn't progress. When I listened to my heart, took breaks as needed, and wrote when I truly felt the call, the muse appeared. Major efforts require copious amounts of patience.

MIX IT UP

Another key in avoiding burnout and/or dropping out is variety. An opera singer doesn't master her art by signing a single aria. She explores all kinds of pieces, even different styles of music. Same goes for becoming more physical. Experiment with a number of different activities—it's better for your mind and body.

REFUTE IRRATIONAL, LIMITING BELIEFS

If you have unrealistic doubts about your abilities, label those doubts as irrational. "I'm not good at anything" is one example of an irrational, self-limiting belief. To counter it, make a list of things you are good at, and post it on your mirror, dashboard, and/or screensaver. Recall concrete examples that dispute any limiting beliefs.

I AM GOOD AT . . .	CONCRETE EXAMPLES
1. _____	_____
2. _____	_____
3. _____	_____
4. _____	_____
5. _____	_____

USE AFFIRMATIONS

While self-affirmations are often ridiculed, research shows that when used properly, they can be helpful (for just one example see L. Legault, T. Al-Khindi, M. Inzlicht. "Preserving Integrity in the Face of Performance Threat: Self-Affirmation Enhances Neurophysiological Responsiveness to Errors." *Psychological Science*, 2012; DOI: 10.1177/0956797612448483). When you write or speak an affirmation about a desired goal, state it in the present tense and be as specific as you can.

(example: I am sitting in my beautiful newly renovated kitchen, appreciating the rich, walnut cabinets and quartz countertops. I feel alive, content, and motivated.)

FIVE EXAMPLES ARE:

1. _____   _____
2. _____   _____
3. _____   _____
4. _____   _____
5. _____   _____

BREAK IT DOWN

Break large projects into manageable pieces. Reward yourself when you've accomplished each step, even if it's simply saying to yourself "Good job!" When I've completed a big project, I always take at least several minutes to "soak it in," appreciating what I've done. After mulching the garden each spring, for example, I sit, breathe deeply, and take a good long look at my gorgeous newly spruced-up flower and vegetable beds. I revel in how good they look. Then I make my long-suffering husband do so, too, while I brag about how much work I just did.

REACH OUT TO COMMUNITY

One of the best ways to find like-minded people is to use your interests as a guide. Join volunteer organizations that work to support goals you are passionate about or take a class in something you love. Better yet, start your own group.

FIND A ROLE MODEL

Pay attention to your role models. Notice what they do. Ask them how they achieved things similar to what you want to accomplish.

ASK A SPONSOR

A "sponsor" is a new buzzword in the business world. Sort of like godparents, sponsors push you to make your dreams come true—but in the process, you also make them look good. In a 2013 *New York Times* op-ed article, Sylvia Ann Hewlett, an economist and business innovator, explained the difference between sponsors and mentors this way: "Mentors act as a sounding board or a shoulder to cry on, offering advice as needed and support and guidance as requested; they expect very little in return. Sponsors, in contrast, are much more vested in their protégés, offering guidance and critical feedback because they believe in them."

CHAPTER 14

Taking risks:
Aim for the moon,
fall among the stars

A former coworker of mine once shared with me that he was a hoarder. He and I worked in different departments but ran into one other at the copy machine or in the hallway. Every now and then we had lunch or coffee together. Having endured tight quarters, the inability to entertain in his own home, and deep shame, he said he really wanted to change his ways. During a walk after lunch one sunny afternoon, he announced out of the blue that he was able to at last clear out his living room. "I even rearranged the furniture," he said, pride clear in his voice. We later toasted the milestone with iced vanilla lattes.

A few weeks later, we ran into one another, each on our way to or from various errands. I wasn't sure what, but something seemed different in my colleague's gait. Or perhaps his eye contact was more direct. "You won't believe what happened this weekend!" Though the hallway's uncharacteristic quiet lent a modicum of privacy, he kept his voice down, but it was clear he was bursting to tell me something.

"What?" I said, smiling back, eager to hear the news.

"I went to the Powderhorn Art Fair," he said, checking to make sure no one else was nearby. "I was just enjoying the weather and looking around, not planning on buying anything. But I fell in love with a painting." At first, he couldn't bring himself to buy the piece, he said. But he kept going back to the artist's stall. "Finally, at the end of the day, I bought it!" I congratulated him.

"I figure this is my reward for all the hard work of getting rid of all that crap," my friend added.

I grinned from ear to ear. "Well, what is this painting like?" I asked.

"I can't describe it," he claimed, a bit too quickly.

"Well, what drew you to it?" I persisted.

My friend was silent. All he could do was shake his head. Then he said, "It's an abstract, and it has a lot of color." That was as specific as he would get.

"Do you have a picture of it?" I finally inquired. He didn't. He then changed the subject, updating me on a conflict he had been experiencing with a coworker. His ploy worked; the new topic distracted me. I remained intrigued, and over the next several months, whenever we ran into each other, I'd ask about the painting. He would mumble a few words about how he was still enjoying it and make some excuse to get quickly back to work. We never went for a walk or shared a meal or coffee again.

When he took a new job on the other side of town, we lost track of each other.

Now I think I see what may have happened. To my friend, the painting was more than just a painting. It was a visual expression of what he considered the best in himself. Chances are he was highly anxious at the possibility of my not liking it. He would have experienced my disapproval as personal rejection—of him, not the painting. He couldn't take that risk. My pressing the issue no doubt scared him off. Looking back, I realize I had unwittingly put too much focus on something that made him feel vulnerable. His inability to share his newly acquired artwork reflected his reluctance to share himself.

"We are constantly given opportunities to become bigger than we are."

The people I interviewed for my happiness videos, on the other hand, allow themselves to be vulnerable. They are all about sharing themselves with others. It's an essential component, in fact, of their true and lasting happiness.

Sitting comfortably in my dining room during his video interview, Dr. Emmons and I explore the intersection of vulnerability, risks, and failing. I ask him what helps people take risks. "It involves being able to accept yourself as fully as you can. Self-derision and self-hatred are so prevalent these days," he says, a hint of sadness in his voice.

"Taking risks is so much easier to do if we have a good sense of our-selves as being okay. If we can really accept ourselves as we are, then failure doesn't hold such a sense of fear," Dr. Emmons states, his hands making circles for emphasis. I am struck by the wisdom of this. If we don't accept ourselves as we are right now, then we won't risk trying to change.

I have one of those "ah-ha" moments. So that's what holds so many of my clients back, I realize. They already feel bad about themselves. If they try and fail, they take it as further proof they're not okay and feel even worse. I think of my former coworker. The purchase of the painting for his newly cleaned-up living room was a big step for this self-proclaimed hoarder. Like most hoarders, he harbored a lot of shame about the way he lived. He couldn't risk sharing any more of himself than he already had.

Accepting themselves as they are allows happier people to be open to change. It's yet another great paradox. In order to make changes, we must accept ourselves first. Without self-acceptance, we can't take risks because what if things don't work out? Our self-esteem would plummet. But when we accept ourselves, as nearly all happy people do, then we won't take failing personally. Our self-esteem remains intact. We're not crushed. (For more on self-acceptance, see Chapter 16: Embracing difference.)

Want to be happier? Learn to accept and embrace all aspects of your-self, including the brave side of you and the fearful side of you. Once you can accept yourself, then test the waters by making change.

"I promise to be fearless."

Take Barry. With the clear fall light streaming in through his large Connecticut living room window, he turns to me and says, "I am largely unbothered by a lot of things. I'm fearless, too." Once again, I am intrigued by his bold statements and want to hear more. "I try not to over-catastrophize. I always say, 'I may not be good at this, but I promise to be fearless about it.'"

As I sit back for another amusing anecdote, Barry describes visiting a diving class taught by his friend, Wayne. Never having learned how to dive, Barry was inspired by the joy and discovery on the students' faces. Moreover, he completely accepted the fact that he was a grown man who did not know how to dive off a diving board. He didn't feel a drop of shame about it.

Undaunted by age or gender, he signed right up. "It was me and eight little girls." With lanky Barry standing nearly six feet, the image of him surrounded by a group of little girls brings a huge smile to my face.

"The best part was this girl's father used to come and watch, and saw me taking the diving lessons. And about the third or fourth class in," Barry gushes, "he signed up for the class, too. So there I was with this dad and all these little girls."

Diving off the diving board for the first time, Barry tells me, "It hurt my head a little, but I was okay. I feel good about it." I like how, with that last part of that statement, he reinforces his own effort. He doesn't just do it and move on without thinking about it. He affirms himself by noticing that the accomplishment feels good. He gives himself credit for taking the leap (in this case, literally). His mental affirmation serves as reinforcement. This is how self-acceptance becomes a reality.

For too many of us, it's a novel idea to tell ourselves we did something well. Perhaps the idea has never occurred to us. And, like any habit, it can be hard to do something new. It takes time and effort to retrain the brain.

Barry emphasizes that he doesn't overdo risk-taking. In fact, he claims he is cautious and measured. I can see that he listens to his intuition. He doesn't push himself beyond his comfort zone. But I also see that he goes to the limit. How? He finds support, takes care of himself, and respects his boundaries.

It's said that optimum human performance occurs when people are neither bored nor overwhelmed. Barry is a master at finding that balance. "I'm the one standing at the very edge of the ledge, looking over. Or I will be the one who will continue inching my way out to see if we can just get a little better view," he boasts. "But I'm actually really careful. If I sense that it's dangerous, I'm not going to do it at all. I'm not reckless."

Barry intentionally takes risks to stretch himself. In doing so, he creates a self-affirming cycle. How so? Finding he can do more than he thought improves his self-confidence, and feeling better about himself helps him take more risks.

"You Have to Stay at It"

Minneapolis filmmaker Ryan has a similar attitude toward taking risks. "You *should* fail at times," he says. In fact, he believes we need to redefine the word failure. "Every time I fail, I see it as a learning opportunity—to improve myself and to get better. The next time I'm going to be better equipped to succeed. It's only a genuine failure if you don't learn from it. It's just a learning opportunity."

Ryan admits he can understand people avoiding taking risks. It's what he did when he was partying and skipping classes before discovering his filmmaking passion. "People want to be comfortable," he says, looking around my office as he searches for words during his interview. "Steady job, income, pay rent, wake up and know they're going to be okay. And that's fine." So he doesn't judge people for their choices. But he also doesn't stop there.

This flourishing 20-something inspires me as he proclaims, "If you want something more out of life, then you're going to have to take risks. Sometimes it's not going to work out, but if you're pursuing something you're passionate about, it's not going to matter." Ryan himself serves as a great example. I greatly admire his confidence, especially since he is so young. Moreover, he is humble and approachable. It is easy to imagine things come easily to Ryan. It's tempting to project only the good onto someone like him and imagine he's never suffered setbacks or rejection.

So when he went on to say, "Every time I've been rejected for a grant, I've never for a moment thought I should do something else," I was taken aback. How could someone as amazing as Ryan ever be rejected from anything? But obviously, even the brilliant, funny, talented Ryans of the world get turned down sometimes. I must admit I find the thought reassuring. Come on, he's young, smooth, accomplished, attractive. If *he* faces rejection, maybe it's okay if I do, too.

"How do you handle it?" I ask. Instead of giving up, Ryan says that he tells himself, "I'm just going to keep going, I'm just going to keep doing it. It's just a small group of people, and I can submit my grant to someone else, and they might all love it. If I don't keep going, then those opportunities aren't going to come. You have to stay at it, every day. If there's something that you want to do, you have to stay at it."

One strategy I've found helpful in building resilience is defining success as *making attempts toward a goal*, not strictly achieving the desired outcome. For Ryan, he might give himself credit for making the effort to *apply* for a grant, regardless of whether he receives it. Reinforcement for trying increases the likelihood that he'll keep at it, even in the face of a setback. This approach also helps one focus on the process versus the result—or to "smell the flowers" as the saying goes.

How do you do stay with something as complicated as filmmaking, I ask Ryan. "You break it down step by step," he tells me. "Most things aren't that difficult. It's just when you look at the whole thing, everything you have to do, that you feel overwhelmed. But that's not how you take on the task. You do it in stages."

In his case, he started small by taking acting classes in college. "I never liked the theater kids in high school," he chuckles, recognizing the irony, "and now I am one." I am charmed by his big, self-deprecating grin. "From the first thing I ever directed, getting together with the actors for the first time to rehearse, it was like, 'This is it. I could do this all day, every day.'" He had found his calling. Today he's one of Minnesota's top up-and-coming filmmakers.

If You Aim for the Moon You'll Fall among the Stars

Some might say Ryan, like other successful people, is "just lucky." In fact, we make our luck. I am reminded of what Barry told me during his video interview about a study he had read regarding luck. "People who perceived themselves to have good luck or bad luck really had no more better or worse luck than anybody else," he recalls. "What they found out is that people who perceived themselves to have good luck did more things and created more opportunities for themselves."

Think about it. Whatever you're after, trying more often—as those who believe they have good luck do—results in more opportunities for success.

"You've got to go out and make things occur, and then every once in a while something good will happen," Barry encourages. "And that sort of breeds itself.

"This is so cheesy, but it struck me at the time and I haven't forgotten it," Barry says, chuckling. "We were in Mystic, Connecticut in some little junk store. I'm sure you've seen those little pillows, they're sort of satiny and they have clever sayings stitched on them. This one said, 'Always shoot for the moon, because even if you miss, you will fall amongst the stars.'

"If we go for it and it's a miserable failure, then A) at least we did it, so no regrets, and B), like, oh, we met so-and-so, that was kind of cool. Or, we learned more about da, da, da. There always are positive outcomes to those kind of things, even if the initial thing didn't work out."

I don't know whether Barry bought the pillow, but the sentiment clearly made an impact on him. In fact, he calls it one of his operating philosophies, and it got him thinking further. "That's another thing I would say. I make mistakes a lot. I think one of the things I've discovered is the difference between making a mistake and failing, because failure is awful. If they were just mistakes, well, we all make mistakes. That's cool." For many of us, the word "failure" is loaded with feelings of shame and self-doubt; whereas the word "mistake" is viewed as a more neutral word, focusing more on the action than on the person's character.

So go ahead, take a dive off that diving board. Sign up for an acting class. Show off your paintings. If you accept yourself, then other people's responses won't matter much. How you feel about your accomplishment, however, *will matter*—and it will feel great.

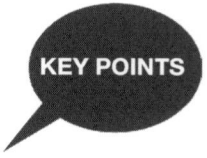

KEY POINTS

- Happier people take more risks and allow themselves to be more vulnerable
- It's easier to take risks when we believe we are okay
- It's possible to take risks and honor our boundaries
- Focus on the process more than the result
- Distinguish between failing and making mistakes; the former may seem terminal, the latter temporary
- People who believe they have good luck try more often, so they appear to have more successes
- Even successful people experience setbacks

PUTTING IT INTO PRACTICE

ACCEPT YOUR FEARS I used to own a copy of the book: *Feel the Fear and Do it Anyway* by Susan Jeffers. Decades ago I lent it to a client (I don't recall whom) who never returned it. I'm not bitter; I figure they need it more than I do. It's been so long, in fact, that I barely remember the book itself at all. But the title has remained with me. What a great concept. It's okay to feel afraid. Courage, of course, is not the absence of fear, but being afraid and doing the right thing anyway. Know you're afraid. Own it. Accept it. Explore it. It may have great messages for you. The idea here is not to let it rule you. Find ways to support yourself through the fear and do what you want to do anyway.

DISCERN RATIONAL FEAR FROM "AVOIDANT FEAR" If a situation is truly dangerous, obviously listen to your gut and protect yourself. Most situations in modern life aren't truly life threatening, however. If your fear is "avoidant"—causing you to avoid what you'd truly like to do, use the strategies below.

GO SLOWLY Start slowly, respecting your boundaries, limits, and capabilities. As Barry said, he doesn't put himself in danger. Yes, there is some risk in diving, but he also reminded himself that he was learning from a professional instructor he knew and trusted, and who was right there. Diving looked like fun. Though he was afraid, he did it anyway.

MAKE IT MANAGEABLE Break large, daunting projects, into simpler, more manageable components. Identify the larger goal, and then record steps you can take to get there.

GOAL:

_____

FIVE STEPS I CAN TAKE TO GET THERE
1. _____
2. _____
3. _____
4. _____
5. _____

DEFINE SUCCESS AS THE ATTEMPT VS. THE OUTCOME
Sometimes things don't work out as we'd like. Reward yourself simply for trying, even if it didn't go as you originally hoped. Focus on what you learned. Think of a time you didn't reach a goal. What did you learn from the experience?

_____
_____
_____
_____
_____

WHAT I'D MOST LIKE TO DO

_____
_____
_____
_____
_____

I WILL SUPPORT MYSELF BY

1. _____
2. _____
3. _____
4. _____
5. _____

MY DEFINITION OF SUCCESS

_____
_____
_____
_____
_____
_____

THE POST-REVIEW

I TRIED

_____

I REWARDED MYSELF BY

_____

I LEARNED

_____

_____

_____

_____

_____

_____

STAY AT IT None of us learned to walk without falling down over and over again. Inevitably, challenges and roadblocks are going to appear. Persistence is key. However, it is good to sometimes see setbacks as opportunities to pause and reflect. You may need a brief break to relax, rest, and recover. Review your priorities. Has your goal changed? Based on what you have learned thus far, what do you want now? This is how you build resilience.

IN THE FACE OF A SETBACK, I WILL

_____

_____

_____

_____

_____

_____

_____

For more on supporting yourself, see the next chapter: Supporting yourself.

PART THREE

Beyond Happy

CHAPTER 15

Supporting yourself:
Exit the highway

While I'm in Michigan visiting family early one winter, Philip invites me to his downtown Detroit workplace for his happiness interview. A converted warehouse, natural light floods the interior, which is decorated in hip, flexible loft/industrial furniture. Several employees dart around accomplishing myriad important tasks, others are fixed to their computer screens, and still others chat informally, seeming to have all the time in the world. Throughout, the place is abuzz with creative energy.

Once he and I are settled in to a back conference room, Philip soon tells the tale of a far different environment. A few years before, just out of college, Philip worked for a high-powered Fortune 500 company in downtown Chicago. He was making close to six figures and dressing to the nines. For many, it would be considered a dream job. Yet Philip was miserable.

"I had no interest in what I was doing," Philip says. "I didn't care about the company and I didn't care about the job." He was bored. The corporation's values in no way inspired him, nor did they align with his own. He felt he had no opportunity for creativity, and he wasn't connected with those with whom he was working. "I was the most unhappy I've ever been."

It's hard to imagine Philip in such a state; now sitting across from this dynamo in his signature jeans and a brown hoodie, he is clearly relaxed and brimming with enthusiasm and positivity. The image of him in such misery a year or so prior is as disconcerting as it is heartbreaking. At the corporate gig, he felt like a cog in a big, impersonal wheel. "I was a little number in a sea of zeroes," he says. He knew he had to do something. Following some soul searching, he made the decision to resign.

"Many people don't understand it. I walked out." I guess I'm not most people; upon hearing this, I'm tempted to lead a cheer. So few people actually do what Philip did: abandon a life that impresses others but that they themselves hate.

How did he do it? First, Philip bravely opened to his internal sensations. He recognized that his pain and angst were messages from within that something needed to change. He reflected on what is really important to him and what he truly wants in life. He realized that being happy was key to his being successful. "Happiness is an anchoring force in my life. I'm almost ridiculously obsessive about the notion of being happy." Philip made the conscious choice to make his personal happiness a top priority by aligning his career with his values. Then he sought "fertile ground," a phrase Philip learned from his dad. Philip considers fertile ground "where we become the most engaged." Trees, crops, and flowers—all essential to life—thrive when planted in fertile soil. The same is true for us. To flourish, we need environments that provide the right nutrients, in this case nutrients that feed our souls. We need settings that provide just the right amount of both challenge and support, that provide opportunities to have an impact on things that matter to us, and that allow us to be who we truly are. None of this was true for Philip in downtown Chicago.

Fast forward a few years, and now Philip is a mover and shaker a few hundred miles to the east. As founder of a multimedia company in Detroit, he is transforming not only the city's image, but also the city itself. "We're not just living in this place. We're redefining it. We once changed the world with the automobile. Who's to say we won't do it again?" It's clear he is now completely engaged.

His enthusiasm is palpable. It's easy to imagine how Philip's passion and positivity breathe life into all his projects. His company's street events, art installations, and merchandise promote the virtues of this often disparaged and much misunderstood city. What most excites Philip, though, is documentary filmmaking. His latest film compares Detroit with Lodz, a city in Poland. Though half a world away, Lodz abounds with eerily similar challenges and opportunities. While the two cultures are very different, both these former manufacturing giants now struggle with dwindling populations and high unemployment—and both are reinventing themselves.

The parallels don't escape me. A young man in a career that didn't fit him is drawn to a city in dire need of transformation—in need of someone like Philip, who was willing to take a chance on it.

Philip found a place that nurtures his happiness, and it is having a huge ripple effect. Philip is now able to transfer his lessons to an entire city.

While Philip's story may make it look easy, we all know making major changes is anything but. Fear of the unknown—of trying something new—is the kind of thing that holds many of us back.

I see this so often in my clients. They're suffering and they know they need to do something different, something big. The second they allow themselves to seriously consider making a change, however, anxiety stops them cold. For some, it's the fear of making a mistake. Others fear losing status. Then there is always the age-old fear of losing money. Such fears prevent many people from recognizing they have options, let alone contemplate making a move. Even highly creative people sometimes forget that there are alternatives. In such a state, thinking often becomes dualistic. When highly anxious, people are often unable to list the benefits a change might bring; they can list only the cons, and no pros.

"What Do You Need to Do to Support Yourself?"

To counter such thinking, I use a key question. To my clients who are facing such fears, I ask: "What do you need to do to support yourself?" This comes from my favorite definition of anxiety, which is "unsupported energy." When we want something important, the desire to get it often makes us anxious. The "What Ifs" are endless: What if we fail?

What if it costs too much? What if we get it and it turns out we don't want it after all? But we forget that the desire to get something is actually energy that motivates us to take action. Our bodies experience that energy in a variety of ways. Anxiety often manifests in physical sensations such as butterflies in the stomach, sweaty palms, and lowered body temperature. The knees might shake a bit, the mouth may get dry, and the heart rate could go up. All these changes are designed to help us fight or flee danger. These autonomic processes enable us to run really fast to escape a bear, but they may not help much when the bear we are facing is whether or not to quit a job. If it were a real bear, all that expenditure of energy would save your life. But when the bear is internal, all that fearful energy can be wasted.

The trick is to harness what's already there. Remember, anxiety is unsupported energy. Find ways to support the energy you naturally have for something you want. This leads to a simple question: What do I need to do to support myself? (Just because it's a simple question doesn't mean the answer or the process of finding it is always easy, of course. But the formula itself is straightforward and easy enough to remember.)

The answer often starts with the breath. When afraid, many of us breathe more shallowly. Taking in deeper breaths interrupts the body's anxiety response and triggers the brain's calming reflexes.

Tightrope walkers, to use an extreme example, learn their sweat-inducing trade by starting with support. Support may come in many forms. Students watch masters for hours. They get expert guidance. Initial lessons are taught on ropes that are close to the ground. As the ropes are raised higher, harnesses and spotters are used to cushion falls. When even higher, safety nets are installed. Only the very advanced perform without a protective safety net.

If you're facing a risk, take a moment and think about how you can start close to the ground. Get some harnesses and safety nets in place. When my dream job turned into a nightmare, I knew I wanted to make a change. How did I support myself? First, I had the incredible blessing

SUPPORT YOURSELF

Anxious? Afraid? Remember, in modern life, most anxiety = unsupported energy. So the formula—while not necessarily easy—is simple. Support yourself.

1. Since most of us breathe more shallowly when anxious or afraid, the first step is to breathe more deeply. Start on the exhalation. Let out more air. This naturally propels the body to breathe in more deeply.

2. Because many of us ignore our body when afraid, the next step is to identify where in your body you are feeling the fear. Scan the body slowly from head to toes. What sensations are you experiencing? There may be butterflies in your stomach, for example. Open up to the butterflies. See how they may shift; they may even disappear just by attending to them! If they don't dissipate, ask your stomach or the butterflies themselves what they are telling you. Get quiet enough to listen for the answer.

3. Identify what messages you may be heeding that you don't truly believe. Do I have the right to be happy? to say no? Dispute any irrational self beliefs.

4. Ask a friend for help. People often isolate when afraid. Talking with a trusted friend can help reveal what you alone can't access. Maybe tell a colleague you're considering taking this risk. Or perhaps invite a friend to come along.

5. Keep asking yourself, "What do I need to do to support myself right now?" The needs are likely to change over time.

of my spouse. Greg's support was critical. After hearing me complain so much about my job, he was as interested in my changing jobs as I was. Second, I reminded myself of times I'd taken leaps of faith before and come out better for it. Third, I told my friends that I was going to resign, because I knew they'd be there for me if and when I hit rough patches. My safety nets included Greg, myself (by way of my history, and reminding myself I can do it), and my friends.

In a culture like ours that so values financial success and image, it can be easy to stay in situations that no longer are satisfying. Many of my clients forget that they have the right to be happy. Had Philip stayed at his job in Chicago, he'd likely be making four times his current income. Through trusting himself, affirming his right to be happy, and planting that happiness in fertile ground, Philip is no longer a little number in a sea of zeros. He's one of the "richest" (read: "happiest") men I know. As he says, "Don't be afraid to exit the highway."

KEY POINTS

KEY POINTS

- Money doesn't guarantee happiness
- Doing what you love brings true wealth
- Anxiety is unsupported energy
- Ask what you need to do to support yourself
- Explore ways you can support yourself to do the things you most want to do
- Place yourself on fertile ground
- Affirm your right to be happy

PUTTING IT INTO PRACTICE

EXIT THE HIGHWAY Philip needed to escape an environment that fed his pocketbook but was crushing his soul. What highway do you need to escape?

_____

_____

_____

_____

_____

_____

TRUST YOURSELF Despite pressure from well-meaning family and friends, Philip trusted his instinct and left a job that made him miserable. List positive decisions you have made in favor of your personal happiness, even if others disagreed.

1._____

2._____

3._____

4._____

5._____

IDENTIFY YOUR RIGHTS Philip believed in his right to be happy. That belief helped him stay on course. It allowed him to take risks that would make his happiness a reality. What rights do you need reminding of? The right to say no? The right to live free of fear or harassment?

I have the right to_____

I have the right to_____

I have the right to_____

I have the right to_____

I have the right to_____

PLACE YOURSELF ON FERTILE GROUND What do you need to make your happiness a reality? Be as specific as possible. Do you need to be in a certain environment? find like-minded people who share your passion? change your current surroundings?

To be happy, I need (1) _____

To be happy, I need (2) _____

To be happy, I need (3) _____

To be happy, I need (4) _____

To be happy, I need (5) _____

DETERMINE THE HOW How I will achieve each of the above needs

1. _____
2. _____
3. _____
4. _____
5. _____

IDENTIFY SUPPORTERS Seeking out the support of family members and trusted friends can make all the difference. Ask yourself, who has always believed in me? To whom can I turn when the going gets rough? Who tells me the truth, even when I may not want to hear it? Who is a good role model for what I want?

1. _____
2. _____
3. _____
4. _____
5. _____

CHAPTER 16

Embracing difference:
Squeaky brakes and sensitivity

Three friends and I nab the last remaining outdoor table at a corner café along Nicollet Mall in downtown Minneapolis. Cars are banned from this idyllic inner-city street; buses, taxis, and bicycles are the only vehicles allowed. Breathing in the stunning early summer day, we sip our iced teas as we await the delivery of our sandwiches and coleslaw. We watch as bikers pedal toward the river and runners pass by on their way to the Greenway, a tree-lined, pedestrian-only corridor connecting Nicollet Mall with the lush and stately Loring Park. Surrounded by friends, drinking in the conversation along with my lemony iced tea, and appreciating the warmth of the sun on my forearm, I feel completely in the moment and happy as can be.

But then I hear it—the screech of a bus coming to a stop. Before I know it, it happens again. Every time one of the behemoths slows, I wince. Geez! Don't those brakes ever get serviced? Am I the only one who cares about noise pollution? Looking around, however, I see that no one else is sticking their fingers in their ears to block out the excruciating, high-pitched, squeaky sound.

I ask my friends if the screeching bothers them. "I don't hear anything except you whining," one deadpans. Our other friend oh-so-helpfully looks at me like I'm crazy. They hear the brakes, all right, but it doesn't bother them. How can it not bother them? To me it's like fingernails on a chalkboard. The afternoon is not ruined, but I'm irritated and distracted each time a bus slows or stops nearby. Can my happiness be so easily marred by screechy brakes?

What's wrong with me? Why am I plagued by something others don't even notice? It's like a curse. I can be perfectly happy doing something one moment and then suddenly I am derailed by an annoying sound, a strong scent, or a shift in the room's temperature. I realize that in these instances, what I feel is shame for being so sensitive, for being so easily upset by such a tiny thing as squeaky brakes.

Fast-forward 18 months and the first hint of an answer comes while Greg and I are on vacation, visiting an aquarium. We watch as dolphins spiral in a huge blue semi-circular tank. At the tank's base stands an interactive display that includes earphones that allow visitors to compare their hearing range to that of dolphins', and to compare an individual's range to the average person's. Greg's hearing range turns out to be about average. Mine, while no match for any dolphin's, is way above average for a human. I hear frequencies most people don't. So that explains the painful bus stops. It's not in my mind, just in my ears.

It turns out that's only part of the story. A few years later, I'm reading a book entitled, *Quiet: The Power of Introverts in a World that Can't Stop Talking* by Susan Cain. She writes about how our culture devalues introverts. I couldn't agree more. Then about half way through, I come upon a concept that changes my world. It's a reference to "the highly sensitive person," and the woman who coined the term, Dr. Elaine Aron. "Highly sensitive people" are more affected by all kinds of stimuli to a much greater degree than most people. And it's not just to high-pitched bus brakes, but aromas, bright lights, even long to-do lists. That sounds just like me! Aron wrote a whole book, aptly titled *The Highly Sensitive Person*. I must have this book! I immediately go online to find it. In the process, I read the book's back cover. "Do you have a keen imagination and vivid dreams? Is time alone each day as essential to you as food and water? Are you 'too shy' or 'too sensitive' according to others? Do noise and confusion quickly overwhelm you? If your answers are yes, you may be a Highly Sensitive Person." I am dumbstruck. All those descriptors apply. Is this book about me? I order it, forking over extra money for overnight shipping (something I rarely do).

When the book arrives the next day, I tear through the packaging and flip to the self-test in the opening pages. "I seem to be aware of subtleties in the environment." Like buses' brakes? Check. "Other people's moods affect me." Oh, yeah. I nearly always seem to sense what those nearby are feeling. "I am very sensitive to pain." I stub my toe in our dining room and the neighbors think I've been attacked by zombies. "I am easily overwhelmed by bright lights, strong smells, or sirens close by." I am laughing now. How many times do I drive Greg batty with my No Overhead Lights rule. Not to mention, I seem to be the only one who can tell when milk is about to go bad. The checklist continues: "I have a rich, complex inner life. I am made uncomfortable by loud noises. I am deeply moved by theater, paintings, films, dance, and music. I get rattled when I have a lot to do in a short amount of time. Being very hungry creates a strong reaction in me, disrupting concentration or mood." Yes, yes, yes, yes, yes!

At last, someone understands me! I'm not alone in my heightened sensitivity! My shame over being so sensitive begins to diminish. I no longer feel like an outsider, and besides, I am learning that sensitivity offers great gifts. According to Dr. Aron, Highly Sensitive People, or HSPs, tend to be more conscientious, are able to concentrate deeply, are highly creative, and are better at spotting errors and avoiding making them. But I, of course, wonder whether HSPs are happier than those who are less sensitive.

I immediately buy more copies of *The Highly Sensitive Person* for family and friends. The book helps all of us understand that being highly sensitive isn't a neurosis or being "overly needy," as I have, at times, been labeled (and as I myself have wondered). Being highly sensitive is actually simply a trait, like having dimples (which I also happen to sport), an attached or unattached earlobe (mine are the latter if you're wondering), or a second toe that's longer than the big one (I'll allow that to remain a mystery). In other words, one is born with this disposition. It is not acquired.

THINK YOU MIGHT BE HIGHLY SENSITIVE?

It's statistically more possible than you might imagine. According to Aron, HSPs make up about 20% of the population. Consider the following questions:
- Do you have a sense that you process or think about things more deeply than many others?
- Do your emotional reactions appear stronger than others'?
- Is it easy for you to feel over-stimulated?
- Do you tend to notice subtleties in the environment that others seem to miss?

If so, you too just might be one of the 1.4 billion HSPs world-wide. For further information, take Dr. Aron's self-test at http://hsperson.com/test/highly-sensitive-test.

Dr. Aron says that HSP brains work a bit differently from others'. An HSP herself, Dr. Aron, writes, "Our nervous systems seem designed to react to subtle experiences, which also makes us slower to recover when we must react to intense stimuli." We are "more aroused by new or prolonged stimulation," explains Aron. The scientific term for it is Sensory-Processing Sensitivity. "What is moderately arousing for most people is highly arousing for HSPs. What is highly arousing for most people causes an HSP to become frazzled," Dr. Aron explains.

Do I ever know frazzled! Whenever I'm at my limit and need down time—or am suddenly starving and have to eat—I unravel. That's why I often sound so frenzied when my blood sugar is low, or why I need to escape to my quiet, darkened bedroom after a wedding reception. This is one of the ways I practice self-care. For HSPs, self-care is vital for our survival.

While it may be easy for HSPs to be moved to tears of joy, it is just as easy for us to lose that joy over unpleasant changes in our environment, both inner and outer.

We HSPs are good at having moments of intense happiness. Our natural sensitivity automatically tunes in to the gorgeous colors of a sunset, senses the change in the air after a rain, and savors the quiet of a cathedral. But I suspect that we have to work a bit harder to stay happy. We may have an advantage, however, in that we are accustomed to making more effort than the average person just to manage in a world built for less-sensitive types. Going the extra mile for happiness seems natural.

ON SELF-TALK

Many of us have a constant running monologue going in our minds. This helps us process our experiences and make sense of the world. Self-talk is the portion of those thoughts that relate to ourselves. While self-talk can be neutral, many of us—often without realizing it—fill our self-talk with subtle or not-so-subtle put downs. That's what I was doing when I thought there was something wrong with me for being more reactive than others to high-pitched sounds. They're not bothered, I shouldn't be either, I might think. If I can't just ignore it, it's my fault. The problem here, of course, is that my friends didn't have to ignore the buses' squeaky brakes. The sounds didn't bother them in the first place. Knowing about HSPs, accepting my difference, and being aware of my self-talk helped me realize I was unnecessarily berating myself. With more awareness, I was able to reassure myself that I'm okay, even if I hear sounds others don't. This isn't to say that self-criticism is always unwarranted or unhelpful. If I've hurt someone, for example, I may need to examine my motivations and change my behavior. In that case "negative" self-talk can be useful. Bringing mindfulness to my thoughts helps me distinguish when my self-talk is helpful and when it's unhelpful. Less of the irrational, critical, unhelpful self-talk helps me feel happier.

Of those I interviewed, only Mia is a full-fledged HSP. She and I meet at our favorite coffee shop just to talk about this commonality. Mia discovered Dr. Aron's book in 1998 when a favorite graduate school instructor recommended it to her. Like me, Mia found it life changing. She too reveled in reading about the fine art of being sensitive. Even among her fellow HSPs, Mia sees herself as someone who is "off the chart sensitive"—endorsing almost all the items on Dr. Aron's checklist. Being an HSP "makes the world really hard," she tells me. Jarring details often distract her. For example, the bright colors the woman sitting near us is wearing tug at her attention. Thanks to her heightened sensitivity, Mia has always felt "a little crazy." Moreover, she confides that it is hard being around others (including her own family) who do not understand how over-stimulation can affect her. Aron's book *The Highly Sensitive Person* helped Mia validate herself as someone who was highly sensitive, not someone who was exasperating, excessively needy, or constantly critical. Best of all, it gave her permission to have her needs met—particularly for downtime. For HSPs, downtime in a quiet setting with little stimulation is as vital as food and water. In Mia's case, taking these needs to heart allowed her to blossom.

Likewise for me. Accepting and honoring my need for quiet has brought about some amazing changes. By modulating my exposure to stimulation, I am much more even-keeled, productive, and yes, happier. Better still, I can stay happy. I have a newfound respect for sensitivity.

Our society is not very supportive of HSPs. The main characteristics of HSPs (sensitive, quiet, caring, gentle) fly in the face of what society values. I still struggle at times with societal pressure ("Be more extraverted!") and internalized homophobia ("Be more macho!"), but I wouldn't trade my sensitivity to fit in. It's who I am. To be able to be moved by the world's beauty is a gift.

While years of being teased for being sensitive may still bear a scar, I can finally accept it for the wonderful thing that it is. If you're not an HSP, you're likely different from others in some other way, or perhaps in several ways. Self-acceptance is essential for all of us. As George Orwell said, "Happiness can only exist in acceptance." So go ahead and call me a sissy. I can beat you in a hearing test any time.

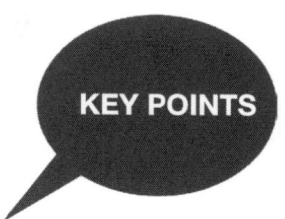

KEY POINTS

- Identify and attend to your needs
- Honoring what you need to recharge your internal batteries is vital to happiness
- Acknowledging your needs and limits can help you be your true self and have authentic relationships
- Accepting yourself for who you truly are not only reduces shame, it also brings more contentedness
- Reframe old definitions of yourself. Aspects that once seemed like liabilities often have hidden advantages. Utilize those benefits, and share them with others

PUTTING IT INTO PRACTICE

IDENTIFY what makes you feel different from others. Often these are attributes that make us feel self-conscious or even ashamed, especially if others ridicule us about them. List those items people tease or ridicule you about.

_____

_____

_____

_____

_____

_____

NOTICE if you judge others for anything listed above.

_____

_____

_____

_____

_____

_____

RECORD your judgmental thoughts of others. Then consider how much you do that same thing.

MY JUDGMENTS OF OTHERS	DO I DO THE SAME THING? IF SO, HOW?
_____	_____
_____	_____
_____	_____
_____	_____
_____	_____

REFUTE Accept that this is where your thoughts currently reside. Begin to gently refute any irrational or untrue judgments. Here, record replacements for the above judgments:

An example: Trish has been living with her partner, Jeremiah, for four years. She feels guilty for calling him a slob. She might write something like this: Jeremiah leaves dirty take-out containers scattered throughout the house, and he rarely picks up his dirty clothes and junk mail, and it drives me nuts! But is calling him a slob a fair judgment? By saying he is a slob, I underscore how neat and tidy I am. But is that really true? I often forget to take out used tissues in my pockets, causing havoc in the washing machine and dryer. And I know Jeremiah hates how the bathroom counter is always wet after I've washed my face. I hate, too, hate both habits in myself. I guess he could call me a slob just as much as I could call him one. But no matter what I do, he never complains. Maybe I'm just as hard to live with as he is. Perhaps I can put up with a few dirty chopsticks in the den and random sweepstakes offers left on the dining room table given all the good things he brings to our household. When I reframe his sloppiness as the actions of someone who works hard and sees his home as a place to relax, I find that I am less judgmental toward both of us. And I can be more accepting of my sloppiness, too.

MY JUDGMENTS OF OTHERS   **REFRAMING THEM**

_____   _____
_____   _____
_____   _____
_____   _____
_____   _____
_____   _____

COST BENEFIT ANALYSIS

List both the costs and the benefits of a need or character trait that you have mixed feelings about.

Trait or Need: _____

COSTS   **BENEFITS**

_____   _____
_____   _____
_____   _____
_____   _____
_____   _____
_____   _____

ACCEPT How can I be kinder toward myself in thoughts, beliefs, and self-talk?

_____
_____
_____
_____
_____
_____

IDENTIFY your needs. What activities help you feel fully alive? Do these activities require that you recharge your batteries?

_____
_____
_____
_____
_____
_____

How do I recharge my batteries?

_____
_____
_____
_____
_____
_____

SEEK COMMUNITY Online or in-person, find like-minded souls—others who share the same trait or interest.

CHAPTER 17

Becoming determined:
Decide. Remind. Decelerate.

It's Tuesday evening, and in my Minneapolis office on the edge of down-town, I am preparing for a favorite aspect of my work: the weekly group psychotherapy session that I facilitate for seven of my clients. To create a circle, I slide a couple of side chairs across the carpet from their usual corner positions; they join two swivel armchairs and a soft, comfy, beige couch around a padded ottoman that serves as a coffee table. I pull the attendance sheet from its home in my middle desk drawer. After adjusting the air conditioning, I make sure the water cooler is full and check that there are plenty of cups and herbal tea selections in the waiting room. As I complete these housekeeping tasks, I have no way of knowing one of my group clients is about to report a major milestone.

DECIDE

Darran had long struggled with severe anxiety. At times his anxiety was so crippling that he felt he could not travel more than five miles from his home. This particular Tuesday, however, a remarkable event occurred. "This morning I was driving to a business meeting," begins Darran. All of us are watching him closely. There seems to be something different about him, a new sense of lightness. "I hit an unexpected traffic jam," he continues, "and in seconds, I am really anxious." He started in with the usual negative self-talk: "I'm going to be really, really late. I'm going to miss the meeting, and my boss is going to fire me. I am such a loser for not going another way. I can't take this."

Highway gridlock can make anyone antsy. But if you've ever experienced clinical anxiety or know someone who has, you know that being trapped in a car at rush hour when you are running late is the last place you want to be when it hits.

The minute Darran felt trapped in his car, his anxiety went into overdrive. At first, he didn't notice that his heart was pounding, his palms were damp with perspiration, and he was barely breathing. What he did notice was that he "began to feel dizzy and light headed." That got his attention—and helped him tune in to the other physical manifestations of his anxiety. It also prompted him to realize that he likely needed to pay close attention to his thoughts.

Instead of ruminating on how awful the traffic was and how he would never make it to his meeting, Darran decided to try something we had talked about many times. While keeping his eyes on the road, he took deep breaths and reassured himself. "This is just anxiety. It will pass," went his internal refrain. Darran looks at us with surprise as he adds, "I became calm." Then his face beams with pride and accomplishment. I can barely keep from applauding.

Darran had made an active decision to make this change—while in the midst of a massive anxiety attack. In that moment, he chose to practice the things he had learned in therapy that would help him through his anxiety. To me, this was nothing less than monumental. After decades of feeling a prisoner to his anxiety and wanting to run from it at all costs, Darran decided to tune in to his body and his thought processes. He consciously slowed down his breathing, which primed his mind to follow suit and stop galloping off with anxious doomsday, self-blaming thoughts. Taking it one step further, Darran told us how he then made another decision to counter his relentless, irrational, negative forecasting. He told himself, "Even if I am late this once, I am a good worker. I'm going to keep my job. I did not cause this traffic. I am a good person."

For someone with clinical anxiety who formerly blamed himself for any setback, no matter how small, this marked amazing progress.

REMIND

No surprise, a number of my happiness subjects use various tools to maintain happiness and keep anxiety at bay. Mia, the Minneapolis therapist, talks about how she uses a technique similar to Darran's to cultivate happiness, which she calls "contentedness." She does this throughout the day, but especially when she's experiencing any difficulties. As she explains it, "I bring my mind to contentedness first by making a really clear choice to do that. There's a way in which I connect with contentedness by reminding myself that it's something I want. I bring my mind to contentedness by reminding myself that it's a choice, and it's something I'm committed to. Frankly, I just prefer it to a lot of other things. So it's having an intention and then reminding myself."

I suspect that reminding herself of her intention to be content is an essential ingredient of her steady, high level of happiness. What does that reminding do? From what I can see, it inclines her brain toward happiness by repeating her goal—"to be content"—over and over again, and following through by making choices that support that intention.

Dr. Emmons has a great way of explaining how powerful making deliberate choices can be, "We need to really begin with our mind," he tells me. "We begin with allowing the mind to calm at least a little bit so that we can be aware of our experiences, but also of our own thoughts and emotional reactions. If we're aware of them, we can choose what we do with them. If we're not aware of them, then we can't do that. We don't have that ability." He pauses and chooses his words carefully. "Awareness is not magic in that it makes everything automatically better. But without it, we just don't have any real leverage. We don't have even the possibility of choosing our reactions to circumstances, of making really conscious decisions and choices. It's got to be there for us to be able to do that."

DECELERATE

One of the simplest ways to become aware of our reactions is to slow ourselves down. Rapid, shallow breathing is a sure sign of lack of self-awareness. Taking slow, deep breaths helps us become aware of our bodies, which in turn takes our focus off our racing thoughts.

When we become more aware of our surroundings and ourselves, it's much easier to make rational, deliberate decisions. In Mia's case, she uses her ability to make purposeful choices to feed her happiness. "There are a lot of things I actually do to help cultivate happiness in my life," she says.

I can see from her arched eyebrows that Mia has more to say. "Such as . . . ," I prompt.

"Sometimes they are pretty goofy, Tom," she says, her voice lowering a bit. "Oftentimes it has to do with beauty. Beauty is one of the things that helps me connect with happiness. So that can be anywhere, right? It can be the pearls I'm wearing," Mia says, running her fingers along her favorite necklace. "It could be having spent time in your beautiful garden or this fabric." She touches the soft woven damask of the couch we're sitting on. "Beauty is really key for me in terms of relating to happiness."

Mia immerses herself in beauty not only via objects, but also in the way she interacts with the world. "I believe that what we extend comes back to us," she tells me. She's referring to the age-old concept of cause and effect, or "what goes around comes around." In other words, every action or thought has an energetic charge to it that will attract similar future thoughts and actions. Positive thoughts tend to create future positive thoughts; negative actions beget future negative actions. "It's a good motivator," Mia says. "And here's another bottom line, I often ask myself, 'What feels good?' Does it feel good to get irritated with the person at the other stop sign who I think should be letting me drive? Or does it feel better to make eye connect and some motion like, 'Please, you go?' Well, the second one. For me, the second one just feels better. So I just keep making choices in that direction. Active choices." If your choices are full of kindness and consideration for others—while simultaneously respecting yourself—then chances are that you will be treated with kindness, consideration, and respect.

When I ask Dr. Emmons what the average, everyday person can do to be happier, he, too, brings up the concept of karma. He had been listening to singer and yoga teacher Gretchen during her in-person videotaping, and he is clearly intrigued by her comments. "Something about her realizing that the present moment was really the result of all the moments that preceded it; all of the things that she had been doing sort of led up to this moment. That is a nice way to think of karma, I believe. What we experience right now is really a result of all actions, all the thoughts, all the things we have done prior to now." He shifts his weight in his chair. "I find that a useful way of framing this notion of how to become happier. Because every day, we're confronted with dozens, probably hundreds of decisions about what are we going to do. If we can bring some conscious awareness to those decisions, virtually any choice that we make can be a choice toward greater happiness." Happiness is a choice; it springs from the decisions we make every day.

In our busy modern lives, with nearly every minute filled with multitasking and overwhelming responsibilities, it's tempting to go on autopilot. We think we'll be more efficient that way, but if happiness is the goal (as many claim it is), we might benefit from being more deliberate.

"I think that it also is really helpful to develop some skill in dealing with unpleasant emotions," Dr. Emmons offers. "To feel your feelings—even when they are not happy, positive, good feelings, this is useful for everyone. We all have times when we're simply feeling bad. We don't like it, but to deny, or escape, or push it away does not help."

"What does help?" I ask.

"Being able to develop ourselves by using awareness," Dr. Emmons calmly replies. (I get the feeling he is highly practiced at this.) "The ability to really experience your emotions, whatever they are, in a deep, complete way so that the emotions can work their way through. We were meant to have emotions. That's why we are wired for being emotional. We need to have emotions—all of them. I think it is a really, really important skill."

I feel chills as I reflect on Dr. Emmons' words. Awareness of emotions helps us develop ourselves. Emotions are our birthright, coded deeply within. Our feelings provide us opportunities to learn, grow, and become better human beings.

Letting ourselves feel all our emotions takes practice—and courage. It's what my group client, Darran, was doing when he noticed anxiety beginning to wrap its foul tentacles around him when he was stuck in traffic. Most of us will do anything to avoid anxiety. From years of experience, however, Darran knew the only way out of it is through it. Resisting the urge to push it away, Darran chose to bravely and fully experience the unpleasant emotion, including all of its physical mani-festations. By slowing down his physical reactions, he was able to make the conscious decision to let his emotions in and see them for what they were—"just fear and anxiety," as he says. While it may seem counterintu-itive, opening to anxiety and welcoming it in like an old friend stopping by for a visit lessens its clammy grip. Darran acknowledged his anxiety, breathed into it, and talked himself through it.

Such awareness and acceptance are the foundations of Buddhism. Mia feels that much of her peace and happiness has come from following its principles. "I've been a practicing Buddhist for 14 years. That means I sit on a meditation cushion," she says with a grin, as if that's obvious. "I have meditation teachers, and I study and practice those teachings of the Buddha. That brings me a profound sense of joy—unlike anything else." Her smile widens. "Those teachings basically say that you are intrinsi-cally well, intrinsically healthy and intrinsically sane. So that's another formula for happiness, right? I think like that, and I've really embodied that. I've heard those things for many years, which is pretty counter-cul-tural, actually." She's spot-on. That's certainly not the message we get from Big Business. They want us to feel in constant need of something to make us feel better—be it an aspirin, a new car, or skinny ice cream. In order to sell us stuff, they make us believe that we aren't good enough. We need more, we need better, we need new.

For Mia, Buddhism is one of the best remedies for modern life. She sincerely believes she is intrinsically fine. "I feel like it's in my cells, and I believe it. And I live from that place that I am and so are you. So the worldview changes, right? When I have a belief that everybody around me is basically good, it allows me to open doorways up to happiness."

How exactly does she do that? I ask her. An example comes to her mind. "So somebody's car alarm went off last night in my neighborhood. I live in a dense city neighborhood, and at one point, I probably would have been rather irritated by it. And then, I remember 'Oh, that person's just wanting to be happy too.' That's what they're going for. They're not trying to annoy me. They're not trying to set off the car alarm for the last three minutes. I think it helps. I assume something better of others when I keep in mind those spiritual principles."

Mia's choices consistently support seeing the good in others because she believes we are all intrinsically good. Yes, one could argue that she is being naïve or unrealistic, but I think not. Every day she Decides, Reminds, and Decelerates. She starts off with the decision to be content. This colors her actions, thoughts, and feelings. When she is confronted with the hassles of everyday life, she repeatedly reminds herself to remain content; she chooses to feel her feelings and actively seeks the good around and within her. What Mia does next is sheer genius: she slows herself down, seeking and then drinking in the beauty around her. Beauty feeds her happiness and restores her inner contentment.

KEY POINTS

KEY POINTS

- Establishing a clear goal to be content and reminding ourselves of it often helps prime the mind to make choices that support it
- Frequent goal reminders help keep us on track
- Calming the mind increases awareness of experiences, thoughts, and emotional reactions
- When we are more aware, we can make better, more deliberate choices

- Experiencing emotions deeply allows them to pass
- Believing that you are intrinsically well and viewing others as essentially good furthers the possibility of happiness

PUTTING IT INTO PRACTICE

DECIDE Make a conscious, deliberate choice to be happy. Elaborate in your own words. Don't be afraid of repeating yourself; here, repetition is your friend, as it can reinforce the idea in the brain and subconscious.

Mia, for example, tells me she brings her mind to contentedness first by making a "really clear choice to do so." In the space below, she might write something such as, "I choose to be content. I want to be content and happy. I remind myself that this is my choice. I commit myself to cultivating contentment. I prefer happiness, peace, and joy."

Today, I choose . . .

_____

_____

_____

_____

_____

_____

REMIND Repeat your goal throughout the day. This type of reinforcement increases the likelihood that you will be able to achieve it. Write your goal on sticky notes and place them in prominent places around the house or your workspace, perhaps even on your car's dashboard. Make it your screensaver.

DECELERATE Slow your reactions down. Breathe. Practice some form of relaxation or meditation daily to help keep your mind calm and increase your awareness. See Chapter 6: Developing mindfulness for more ideas.

FEEL Our emotions provide information. They can lead to wisdom we can get nowhere else. When strong emotions arise, breathe into them. Support yourself with your breath and your mind; remind yourself you can handle this. You've faced difficult emotions before; you can do so again. Notice what is happening in your body. What are these physical sensations telling you? Why is this emotion here now? What is its sacred message? I've seen it time and again with clients, friends, and within myself. If we stay with our feelings long enough, inevitably we come to a new understanding.

CHOOSE Utilizing your increased awareness, make active choices throughout the day that support your goal. Restate your goal, and record action steps that will take you there. For most of us, happiness comes when we connect with others, our passions, and ourselves. For more on this, see Chapter 2: Defining Happiness.

Three examples:

1. GOAL: Make more friends

ACTION: I will take a class on something I am passionate about (be specific)

2. GOAL: Be kinder to myself

ACTION: I will become aware of those times when my self-talk turns cruel and stop saying things to myself that I would never say to anyone else. I will imagine I am talking to a dear friend. What would I say to him instead?

3. GOAL: Explore my passions

ACTION: Set time aside in my calendar to have "a date with my passion," be it kayaking, water color painting, going to museums, bike riding, fishing, bird watching, attending sporting events, or practicing piano

1. GOAL: _____

ACTION: _____

_____

_____

_____

2. GOAL: _____

ACTION: _____

_____

_____

_____

3. GOAL: _____

ACTION: _____

_____

_____

_____

ASK yourself which feels better—aggravation or kindness? Like Mia, for example, to be irritated at the other drivers, or to extend courtesy and allow the other to go first?

_____

_____

_____

_____

_____

BELIEVE/REINFORCE As Mia suggests, live from the belief that you are intrinsically healthy and sane. Make "I am intrinsically healthy and intrinsically sane" a mantra or self-talk. Write it in your own words here, then transfer it to sticky notes and place in prominent places, or use as your screensaver.

_____

_____

_____

_____

_____

_____

VIEW OTHERS AS BASICALLY GOOD Seeing others as acceptable, decent human beings also brings peace.

CHAPTER 18

Aligning your values:
The Circle of Passion

When I'm in Chicago for a friend's wedding, fitness trainer Tracy invites me to his home, a charming Victorian walkup, for his video interview. He's just finished teaching an evening class. We both grab a bottle of water and take a seat in his chic living room, he on the couch, and I on the adjacent armchair. After catching up on small talk, we explore what happiness is to him and how he maintains it. It turns out these lessons were hard won.

With his boyish good looks and joyful, optimistic presence, it's hard to imagine that Tracy was once miserable. "I was a ridiculously unhappy person," he tells me. "I was always looking for accolades. I wanted a pat on the back. I wanted recognition." Who hasn't felt similarly? Looking cool and being popular or sought after can be irresistibly seductive. Feeling wanted and connected to others are, after all, basic human needs. But when they come at the expense of our core values or our passions, trouble inevitably follows. What we love to do should not be contingent upon outside praise. When our need for approval is too strong, we can be unable to even consider, let alone discover, what is most important.

This is precisely what Tracy experienced. His need for approval blocked him from knowing what he himself most valued and enjoyed. "I lived my life from a very fear-based standpoint for a long, long time," he

FULL HEART LIVING

says. My heart goes out to him as I hear the pain and regret in his voice. "There were probably many different things that I was afraid of," Tracy continues, "fear of failure and fear of not being accepted were probably biggest, especially during my teenage years when I felt like an outsider not really fitting into any particular group of people. I felt I was on this spinning wheel of nothingness."

To overcome his fears, Tracy focused on becoming a "success." In junior high and early high school, he excelled at sports, playing on a number of teams and reveling in the resulting accolades. His need to appear successful, however, got in the way of trying to figure out what he truly wanted to do. Initially, he thought he wanted to be a medical doctor, but changed his mind and decided he wanted to work in music, perhaps as a music teacher. Then the acting bug hit. "I decided I wanted to be an actor. I went to a conservatory style program for my BA and pursued being an actor," Tracy says. Soon after graduation, "I got lucky and landed a part in a made-for-TV movie," Tracy tells me. When the filming was completed, he started the process of auditioning again. After months of no acting work, Tracy reluctantly admitted he had hit a dry spell and, low on cash, needed to find work in another industry. Unlike many actors who take jobs that are easy to quit, Tracy took an office job with a law firm. It paid the bills, and he found that he liked the work and loved the people.

As the years passed, Tracy realized that acting wasn't what he wanted. "Trying to be an actor, trying to make a living being an actor, wasn't fun anymore," says Tracy quietly. "I stopped auditioning and stopped thinking of myself as being an actor. Many of my acting friends couldn't believe that I could make that decision. To be honest, considering that it simply wasn't fun anymore, the decision really wasn't very hard to make."

Fast forward a few years, and Tracy started volunteering for his daughter's soccer team. He had always loved being physically fit—it had been one of his passions. And coaching his daughter's team led him to find another one: he loved working with children. He realized he truly wanted to be a coach and work with children to help them feel more confident in how they move

212

their bodies—whether for sports or just everyday life. Eventually, he went back to school and earned an advanced degree in kinesiology. Today, Tracy is a beloved and highly sought-after fitness teacher and coach.

Tracy sits up straighter as he recalls a story about an elementary school student a few years back. "She was very shy and reserved, not a bad mover, but not into sports. After eight weeks, she had all these benefits." Perhaps her greatest gain was feeling more confident and comfortable in her own skin. "Months later, her mom ran into me," Tracy beams. "'You won't believe what happened,' the mom said. 'My daughter came home from school and said, "Mom, I played flag football on the playground."'" Pride clear in her voice." I hear it in Tracy's, too.

Hearing this reminds me of the younger Tracy who searched so hard for accolades, but if he found them, they didn't ring true. The praise from his student's mother hit home. He felt deeply, sincerely appreciated. Possibly even better, he felt appreciated for doing something that really matters to him and that also helps others tremendously. Tracy's true, core values were finally affirmed.

Sometimes it takes fear and failure to point us toward our real passion. Often the fear of not getting approval or of disappointing someone keeps us from doing what we truly love, which is connecting with people who share our passions.

Happiness is a Three-Legged Stool

In my work as a life coach and therapist, and through my video interviews, I have learned that the foundation of happiness is comprised of three key components:
   1) Connecting with yourself in a meaningful, heartfelt way
   2) Connecting with others—being part of a community you care about and that cares about you
   3) Engaging in activities you are passionate about

One of the beautiful things about finding your passion is that it inevitably leads to creating better connections with yourself and with others. I like to call it the "Circle of Passion."

Why is it sometimes challenging for people to discover what they love? Maybe it's simpler than we think. As children, we are naturally drawn to certain things. Some find sports captivating, while some are enthralled by art or music. Still others are fascinated by animals, the outdoors, storytelling, or cars. Whatever the area of interest, problems arise when those pursuits aren't supported. Friends, family, teachers, coaches—anyone with even a little bit of authority can squash a child's dream. If we are told that we are "not good enough" or "don't have talent" or "can't handle the pressure," the resulting shame can be debilitating. Some people believe that these words mean that they chose the wrong activity. In extreme cases, the person ends up despising the activity itself.

UNCOVERING CORE VALUES

How do we go about finding activities and/or work that we can be passionate about? Some people seem blessed to have come into the world never doubting their heart's desire. Others find it more elusive. Conventional wisdom says to search your heart, but that can be challenging. We often value so many things that it can be hard to tell what really resonates deep down within us.

One way to begin exploring what you might love to do is to take a close look at the people you admire. What qualities do they possess that you admire? How do they embody those values? Chances are, their values align closely with yours. Explore those values and then ask yourself what activities/work/interests line up with those values?

Told that what they love to do is "frivolous" or "won't make any money," many bury their passion and do what is "expected" of them. Some people seem to acquire what we might call "passion amnesia," forgetting they ever had any interests or passions. This happens to many of the people who come to me for psychotherapy. Often these folks have no idea what might make them happy. They are convinced that they have no passions and nothing they do truly matters. They often feel resigned, paralyzed, and apathetic. They're convinced they're alone, that no one else hurts as they do, or that others can't understand them.

A client of mine, Jerry, had a longstanding passion for singing. As a small boy watching old musicals on TV, he was transfixed by the power of the songs to move him so deeply. He knew that's what he wanted to do with his life. When he grew a bit older, after much begging and pleading, his parents paid for a handful of voice lessons. But his voice teacher insisted he learn to sing only classical choral music. For a while, he practiced his favorite songs from musicals on the side, belting them out in the shower every morning. But his father complained about the "racket," his brothers teased him, and his mother simply sighed and ignored his "singing phase." No surprise, Jerry stopped singing.

Many years later, as an adult now firmly established in another profession, Jerry decided to try again. He signed up for an intensive three-week musical theater class. At the first class, he was bursting with nerves and enthusiasm, but his heart fell when he realized he was the oldest student in the group. Worse, the other students all knew each other and didn't have the time or inclination for a new, more "mature" friend. Things got worse when the teacher required they first work on opera arias. Opera was way out of his league. Throughout the course, forced to do things he wasn't truly ready for, Jerry felt more and more overwhelmed and unsupported. He even overheard an arrogant fellow student making cruel remarks about his singing voice.

Yes, there were some good days, such as when he worked on songs from the musicals he loved. But by the end of the workshop, he felt depleted and depressed. Reaching a new low, Jerry again stopped singing.

Soon thereafter, Jerry came to see me for psychotherapy. In listening to his story, I realized that he had unwittingly stumbled into a situation that replicated what had happened to him in childhood. Again, he found a teacher who wanted him to sing his way, again he was made fun of, and again he felt isolated and alone. In time he realized that the emotional patterns of victimizing, teasing, and ignoring, which were laid down in his childhood, were like ruts in a road that he automatically slipped into. But just because those ruts were well worn didn't make them true. Nor did it mean he couldn't take an alternate route.

When he talked about music, Jerry was transformed. Leaning forward, the very tone of his voice lifted and became more melodic, as though he unconsciously started to sing. It was as if his whole body couldn't help but rise up, just in talking about singing. I could see his whole body bursting with energy, and he seemed to come alive. I encouraged him not to give up what was clearly so life giving, and I suggested he find a teacher with whom he felt safe—who could help him connect to his need to sing what he wanted and in the way he wanted—and to find a group of people who cherished musical theater as much as he did. Jerry agreed. I coached him to approach this project one step at a time. First he asked around and got the names of several voice teachers. He interviewed each by phone and even checked references. He settled on one who specialized in musical theater. After a year of lessons and mentoring by his voice teacher, he felt confident enough to join an amateur theater company. He started slowly, doing stage crew work. He met a lot of people and found he connected with many of them. With their encouragement, he tried out for small singing parts. Within in a few years, Jerry realized a lifelong dream he almost didn't dare let himself have: he sang the lead in a musical. It was even better than he imagined, because he was now good friends with the other actors and crew members.

If doing what we love makes us happy, then doing what we love in spite of setbacks, conflict, and bad luck makes that happiness all the sweeter. Perhaps that is why comeback stories warm our hearts and give us hope. People who have had to really struggle to find their passions and follow them often are the ones who are there to help others with theirs.

Tracy, who himself had some terrible athletic coaches growing up—critical and demeaning, and anything but emotionally supportive—values emotional support and works to provide it for his student athletes. "If I can be that person who believes in them, then I can give them that support. They may not get it at home, and they may not get it in school." The emotion in Tracy's voice gives me chills, and it's clear how much doing this work means to him. I know that his passion and commitment, combined with his non-threatening, easy-going nature, make Tracy uniquely able to provide such support in abundance.

His enthusiasm, in fact, is infectious. "I believe you can do this," he tells his students, and it works! "I've seen miraculous improvements in their opinion of themselves," Tracy tells me, "what they thought they could do, their ability to overcome fears and become risk takers."

In addition to finding a way to help others through an activity he loves, it seems to me that being a coach has enhanced Tracy's sense of community. He feels valued, wanted, and needed. When you find what you love to do and do it, you are naturally drawn to finding others who love it, too. Community fosters happiness and encourages it to grow.

Sitting across from Tracy, in his black warm up pants and matching shirt replete with his own coaching logo, I am struck by how comfortable Tracy is in his skin. He clearly feels no need to impress others. He doesn't have to. He's okay just as he is. "The thing that I like about my life now," he tells me, "is I feel I have a purpose. There is something important for me to do that makes a difference."

KEY POINTS

KEY POINTS

- Three key components of happiness:
   1) Connecting deeply with yourself
   2) Connecting with others
   3) Engaging in activities you are passionate about
- Exploring our passions leads to creating better connections with ourselves and with others, and often vice versa: the more connected we are with ourselves, the more likely we are to pursue our passions. This is the "Circle of Passion"
- Finding community, connecting with others, and embracing passions supports the development of the true self

- Happy people's actions are in harmony with their values
- Bringing others happiness produces happiness in oneself (and vice versa: being happy ourselves often inspires others to be happy)
- Doing what you love in the service of others further heightens happiness

PUTTING IT INTO PRACTICE

SEARCH YOUR CHILDHOOD

What did you love to do as a child?

_____
_____
_____
_____
_____
_____

When you were young, how did you respond when people asked, "What do you want to do when you grow up?" or more commonly, "What do you want to be when you grow up?"

_____
_____
_____
_____
_____
_____

SEARCH YOUR DREAMS AND PASSIONS

What do you most enjoy doing now?

_____
_____
_____

_____

_____

_____

What do you still dream of doing?

_____

_____

_____

_____

CLARIFY VALUES

1. Circle your top 15 values from this list. So you're forced to not over think your selections, set a timer for a maximum of five minutes.

Community	Leadership
Intellectual status	Status
Serenity	Personal tranquility
Competition	Fast-paced work
Engagement	Actualizing my potential
Personal development	Creativity
Involvement	Location
Sophistication	Decisiveness
Job tranquility	Loyalty
Cooperation	Supervising others
Knowledge	Democracy
Order	Respect
Stability	Achievement
Conformity	Financial gain
Working alone	Physical challenge
Solitude	Getting promotions and advancing
My country	Freedom

Pleasure	Security
Adventure	Ethical practice
Friendships	Merit
Power and authority	Financial gain
Affection, love and caring	Excellence
Personal Growth	Nature
Privacy	Wisdom
The arts	Expertise
Having a family	Fame
Public service	Time freedom
Health and fitness	Effectiveness
Purity	Efficiency
Challenging problems	Meaningful work
Helping other people	Truth
High-quality	Commitment
Fast living	Influencing others
Change and variety	Reputation
Helping society	Competence
Having quality relationships	Working under pressure
Having good character	Excitement
Honesty	Ecological awareness
Recognition	Market position
Close relationships	Independence
Taking care of others	Accountability
Money	Religion
Inner harmony	Spiritual practice
Serenity	_____
Responsibility	_____
Integrity	_____

2. Of the 15, cross out five. Again, set a timer. This time, give yourself a maximum of two minutes.

3. Now give yourself one minute to whittle the list further to five.

4. And one more minute to eliminate two.

5. Write the three remaining values here.

_____ _____ _____

ASSESS I am currently living those values by

_____

_____

_____

_____

_____

ASSESS I am currently NOT living those values by

_____

_____

_____

_____

_____

IDENTIFY Where do you feel part of a community?

_____

_____

_____

_____

_____

EXAMINE How does your community support you in living your values?

_____

_____

_____

_____

_____

EXAMINE How does your community encourage you to ignore or violate your values?

_____

_____

_____

_____

_____

DETERMINE your next step. What I will do to bring my actions more in accordance with my values

_____

_____

_____

_____

_____

COMMIT I will begin _____(insert date— HINT: make it today!) by taking this concrete action:

_____

_____

_____

_____

_____

MAKE A DATE WITH YOURSELF Every three months for the next year, mark in your calendar dates to spend time to review your progress

REVIEW What are my life goals?

_____

_____

_____

_____

How well do my goals align with my values?

_____

_____

_____

_____

_____

DETERMINE your next step. What I will do to bring my goals more in accordance with my values . . .

_____

_____

_____

_____

_____

COMMIT I will begin _____ (insert date— make it today!) by taking this concrete action:

_____

_____

_____

_____

_____

REFLECT How I bring happiness to others

_____

_____

_____

_____

_____

What I can do to bring more happiness to others

_____

_____

_____

_____

_____

COMMIT I will begin _____(insert date—make it today!)
by taking this concrete action:

_____

_____

_____

_____

_____

CHAPTER 19

Overcoming shame:
Life is a painting

Could you be happy if you didn't work in the field of your choice? Could you be happy if you were up to your ears in debt? How about if you had a serious illness. Could you be happy then? Despite a low-paying job, thousands of dollars of debt, and a major mental illness, my interview subject Jenn is happy. This is even more extraordinary because not too long ago, Jenn used to "have it all"—a high-power, well-paying executive position, a long-term relationship, and a beautiful newborn son. "I did all the right things," she reflected. "We bought the house, bought the cars, took the vacations."

How did this all come about? Sitting back in her avocado retro chair in her living room, surrounded by her many sculptures she made out of found materials, Jenn tells me how she woke up one morning, and felt "different." "Everything was a heightened sense. I couldn't think straight," she says. It was as though overnight and without warning, her body completely and dramatically altered. Her mind and energy were accelerated. She felt she couldn't stop moving, pacing, thinking. She couldn't focus and couldn't go to work, she tells me, adding, "All I could do was art." It was her first manic episode. She saw a doctor and was diagnosed with bipolar disorder (what used to be known as manic depression).

Bipolar disorder is marked by episodes of extreme mood swings, from mania to depression, with little warning and usually no clear "precipitating event." During the manic phase, it is not uncommon to have racing thoughts, talk very fast, and behave impulsively. When the mood shifts to depression, concentration is often impaired and memory and decision-making skills may be compromised. Thoughts can turn suicidal. Desperate for a means to cope or escape, many turn to alcohol and/or other drugs. Hence, chemical abuse or addiction is common with bipolar disorder.

After a six-week medical leave from work, Jenn was informed that her position had been eliminated. The ostensible reason: the organization needed to cut expenses. Jenn suspects her mental illness was the true cause.

Unrelated to her bipolar disorder, she and her partner split up soon after. "We just grew apart," Jenn tells me matter-of-factly. The two continue to get along well, however, and to co-raise their son. "We're so great together with him."

In just a few short months, Jenn was without a partner, a job, and a way to pay her bills. Soon the debts mounted, and she found herself under a mountain of expenses. Within two years, the city put a levy on her bank account because she couldn't pay the taxes on her home. Here, Jenn becomes sheepish. "I have always paid my mortgage," she says. But now she could barely afford food or rent. "I was completely out of money, living here with my son."

It was the lowest point in her life, and Jenn felt she was without options. Her illness made working impossible, and she didn't want to tell her friends what was happening. Desperate, and abusing alcohol, she seriously contemplated taking her life. She almost did, but luckily a friend intervened. Two days later, she learned that another friend had killed herself. On the day of the funeral, Jenn took a deep, unflinching look at her own situation. On behalf of her late friend, her son, and herself, Jenn made a silent promise: "I'll never drink again."

Soon after quitting drinking, her mind beginning to clear, Jenn had an inspired idea. She could raise funds by selling her belongings. She invited all her friends to an estate sale, telling them she needed to raise money for rent.

The day before the scheduled sale, her friends started stopping by. One friend bought Jenn's two favorite things, her record player and her bike, and said she'd pick them up later. (Of course she never did.) Some gave her money to "rent" her movies. Others hired her services as a photographer.

Then friends of friends began coming. By the end of the weekend, probably a hundred people came by. With many of them, Jenn did something extraordinary. She told them the full story about what had happened to her. Jenn leans forward and fixes her eyes on mine, saying, "I got to sit down with each one of them and tell my story. Then they felt free to tell their story. And we connected."

By telling them the truth about her illness and her present predicament, Jenn freed her listeners to tell her their "real" stories. Her willingness to be vulnerable allowed others to lower their guard and talk about things that we rarely talk about: our failures, our low points, our bad decisions.

RELEASING SHAME

Is there something you're ashamed of? Something you've never shared with another living soul? Maybe something you can only barely admit to yourself? That kind of shame can wreak havoc psychologically. Conversely, bringing such secrets out into the open with trusted others can bring great peace, freedom, and even joy. Releasing the burden of secrecy leads to greatly enhanced connections, with self and others. Opening to others helps us open to ourselves and often allows them to open up to themselves and to us. Find someone you can trust. Open up. Share your truth.

"Putting the Truth out There Helps Connect You to Other People."

The weekend of her estate sale, Jenn's life took a huge turn for the better. As she puts it, "I saw this sense of community, and it's carried on since then. It's such a part of my happiness. Putting the truth out there helps connect you to other people."

Because of her bipolar disorder, Jenn feels unable to return to her former work as a director and manager. "My mind won't let me," she says. Instead, she has a job that pays minimum wage. But she is proud of being able to work again. "I stand on my feet all day for nine dollars an hour, yet banks and credit card companies are threatening to garnish my wages. They're putting judgments on me," she says.

Then she shifts her weight in her chair and looks directly at me. "At some point I had to throw my hands up," she says. "I basically just had to let go. It's really hard, because I don't like to owe people money. One of these days I am going to pay it all back," she says, a determined expression settling on her face. "In the meantime, I'm going to be happy." I am stunned when I hear her say this. How can she choose to be happy after all the hardships she has encountered? Her answer amazes me. "I had to forgive myself," she says quietly.

Jenn realized she couldn't change the fact that she has bipolar disorder. She can't undo the spending that led to her debt. She can't force herself to work at higher paying jobs she can no longer manage. Instead, she forgives and accepts herself as she is now. This is a vital step. To really be happy we need to forgive and accept ourselves for who we truly are, warts and all. Unfortunately, many of us can't bear to look at the warts until a misfortune makes them only too visible—like Jenn's illness, lost job, and resulting bankruptcy.

Jenn's face brightens as she tells how raising her son, Owen, also has inspired her. "I completely changed with Owen. Allowing him to be himself is a top priority. He's a princess boy, and he likes to wear dresses. As a result, I've let myself be who I am. He's taught me so much. It's okay to be who you were born to be. It's okay for you to live your truth."

In the past, Jenn was extremely feminine; her hair was long, and she wore dresses. As with Owen, she allows herself to explore the full gender continuum. Now her head is shaved, and she almost always sports a driving cap and a wide tie. She doesn't identify as male or female, but somewhere in between. "I don't want to lose myself again. I've discovered who I am inside, and I'm living that. That contributes to my happiness."

I Need to Be Who I Truly Am

I'm reminded of another friend of mine, and not just because this person is also beyond the gender binary. When he turned 30 years old, he wrote to tell me he was changing his name. "I'm calling myself Alison now. I've known for years, as long as I can remember in fact, that I was born into the wrong body. I've tried to hide it, squash it, pretend it wasn't there, tried to pray it and even drink it away. I hated myself for a long, long time. I've tried to 'be a woman on the side,' like some sort of weekend hobby. But I can't go on like that any longer, torn and hiding, going back and forth. I need to be who I truly am, all the time," she wrote.

I was honored to be one of the first to know that she was making the transition to claim her true self and live life as a woman. It's one of the most harrowing journeys I can imagine. Flying in the face of societal norms and coming out as transgender takes great courage.

What impressed me in listening to Alison's story was the role community had played in making it happen. Her journey started alone, at the library. She tucked herself in a corner and read everything she could find on transgender experiences. Becoming braver, she soon turned to the Internet, exploring online transgender forums. Knowing she wasn't alone took the edge off her self-loathing. In time, her confidence bolstered, but still trembling with fear, she drove across town and somehow managed to make her way through the maze of hallways to a corner room on the third floor of an old church to attend a transgender support group. This was the first time she'd met another transgender person face-to-face. "Once I stepped inside, I was so relieved," she told me. "Finally, I was meeting face-to-face with people I could relate to and who could relate to me. You can't imagine what that did for me," she wrote. "I could finally breathe! I was accepted for who I truly am! I was overcome by so many emotions. I couldn't help it. I actually wept in a room full of strangers!"

I asked Alison what they talked about. While occasionally they might share resources, she told me, such as where to buy makeup and shoes and where to go to get your nails done, the vast majority of the time was spent talking about how to live in a world that is only just beginning to understand, accept, and embrace our transgender siblings.

After years of feeling alone and full of doubt and questions, those weekly meetings were Alison's first real experience of being in a community where she was surrounded by a sea of love and acceptance. It was this supportive community that helped to heal Alison's wounds. Self-love and acceptance began to seep into Alison's very core. In time, Alison was struck not only by the similarities of those in the room, but how much they loved one another despite so many differences. "There were people there of every race, religion, and class," she told me. "Some aren't into hair and makeup at all, which perplexed me at first. Others watch football every Sunday, just like me!" Knowing she had the support of this community that embraces similarities and differences, Alison was eventually able to reveal her true identity to her family, friends, and coworkers.

In fact, her two siblings accepted Alison's new identity with open arms. "They just want me to be me. And I can tell they want to remain an active part in my life, no matter what I wear or look like," says Alison. Her mother had a different reaction. Flummoxed, not knowing what else to say, her mom urged Alison to lose weight so she would look more "feminine." Demonstrating remarkable compassion, Alison accepted this veiled slam as an indication of her mom's anxiety and ultimately as an expression of love. When we are overwhelmed, it's not uncommon for us to resort to ingrained cultural conditioning, which is just what Alison's mother did. But Alison was not buying it. "If I'm not going to succumb to pressure to be a gender I'm not comfortable with, I'm certainly not going to adhere to society's unrealistic body standards!" Alison said with her keen intelligence and characteristic self-assurance.

Claiming her true identity, sharing it with others, spending time with people who accept her for who she truly is—a football loving, woman-born-a-man—Alison now lives the life she believes she was meant to live.

The Masterpiece

Like Alison, Jenn, too, found that sharing her true self led to an increased sense of freedom. Buoyed by the support of her friends' selflessness, rescuing her from the brink of homelessness, she was able to further act in ways that reflect her true self. For Jenn, that means making art and dressing in masculine clothing. It also means being able to engage in authentic conversations with people. "I wake up in the morning and I think, How many people am I going to make smile today? Or how many people am I going to engage in conversation? I'm going to smile with them. I'm going to be inspired with them. I go to work thinking, This is going to be a good day."

Jenn takes a sip of her tea. She is reflective for a moment. "It probably took me losing almost everything to get to this point," she says. But what she gained is priceless. She learned that peace and happiness come when you choose to make your happiness a priority. "I'm in control of my happiness, and I have to get there, even if it means I can't pay my bills. It's okay to live your truth."

It took several misfortunes for Jenn to wake up to her true self. In 12-step programs, this is called "the gift of desperation." We can easily become conditioned to the daily circumstances of our life. I suspect this is a survival mechanism; we adapt to survive, failing to register how discontented we are. It often takes misfortune—illness, job loss, relationship break-up, financial set-back, death of a friend or family member—to wake us up to how unhappy we actually are. While it may be hard to see while you are going through it, there is a silver lining in the storm cloud. We then have the opportunity to claim our true, whole, perfectly imperfect selves.

As Jenn so exquisitely puts it, "I view my life as a painting. Each brushstroke represents a moment in time. At the end of my life, I want to have a masterpiece. Little by little, it just gets more beautiful."

KEY POINTS

KEY POINTS

- "Having it all" doesn't guarantee happiness, but being true to yourself might
- Sharing our stories connects us with others
- Divulging our pain inspires others to do the same
- Desperation can breed ingenuity and lead to community
- One can be happy while experiencing conditions that society disparages
- Accepting yourself and your circumstances fosters contentedness

PUTTING IT INTO PRACTICE

IDENTIFY What is not quite right in your life right now? What are you struggling with or ashamed of?

_____
_____
_____
_____
_____
_____

IDENTIFY Three trusted friends with whom I could share this truth:

_____   _____   _____

SHARE Consider how you could share your story with one of those three friends. If that seems undoable, consider seeing a psychotherapist.

WRITE A LETTER TO YOURSELF If there are things you struggle to let go of or forgive yourself for, write about it. Ask yourself how you would feel toward someone else in that situation and what you would say to that person. Say those things to yourself in letter form.

Dear _____[insert your name],

_____

_____

_____

_____

_____

_____

_____

_____

_____

_____

_____

_____

_____

_____

_____

_____

_____

_____

_____

_____

DEFY THE NORM Jenn allows herself and her son to express themselves in dress and behavior counter to cultural gender norms. What have you held back doing or being due to cultural norms, what others might think, or how others may judge you?

_____

_____

_____

_____

_____

_____

SUPPORT YOURSELF What would I need to do to allow myself to experiment with going against the norm?

_____

_____

_____

_____

_____

_____

IDENTIFY Events from the past that still bother me

_____

_____

_____

_____

_____

_____

EXPLORE What I need to do to let go of them

_____

_____

_____

_____

_____

_____

DETERMINE People in my life who allow me to be who I am

_____
_____
_____
_____
_____
_____

INVESTIGATE How I can spend more time with them

_____
_____
_____
_____
_____
_____

CONSIDER Things I've always wanted to do but held back from doing

_____
_____
_____
_____
_____
_____

ESTABLISH What would I need to do to make those things happen

_____
_____
_____
_____
_____
_____

CHAPTER 20

Stepping into full heart living

Looking back on this happiness project, from video to book, it's striking how my perspective has changed. I used to look at my life as simply making it from one milestone to the next, some of them good, some not so good. For instance, I had my dream job, and it turned sour. Following months of unhappiness, I took a huge leap of faith and quit. Painful as it was, I allowed myself to fully experience the resulting grief. This mourning period helped me realize that I had somehow misplaced my long-lost love of performing. I started working in local theater productions. Another big milestone was setting up my own private therapy practice. In time, I found myself becoming happier. Yes, I had lost my dream job, but I had reclaimed parts of myself that bring great joy.

How could so much pain give rise to so much happiness? I started studying happiness, and soon I was teaching classes about how to bring greater happiness into our lives. The more I learned and the more I shared what I was learning, the more energized I became. I decided to go further and interviewed some exceedingly happy and very wise people. I was amazed to see that the insights I gained and the lessons I applied had a huge impact on my own life. I found myself growing happier and wiser in the company of these exceedingly happy yet otherwise ordinary people.

I saw how my interviewees live with their full hearts. Their hearts are open to themselves and others. Doing things they love, they follow their hearts in choosing activities. They express gratitude from the heart. They take good care of themselves. They stay in the present moment. They give to others. They are real, live examples of what loving oneself and others can do.

"It is only with the heart that one can see rightly."
~Antoine de Saint-Exupéry

Early on, it occurred to me that the people I interviewed make different choices than most people do when it comes to ensuring their lives are happy. Consequently, the original title of this book was *Choosing Happiness: Conversations with the Happiest People I Know*. While it's true that their choices set them apart, it wasn't until I was deep into the writing that I had an epiphany. What my interviewees were telling me is so much more than the specific choices they make to be happy. Their wonderful stories spoke of a synergy of the whole, beautiful gestalt that makes up their beautiful, full lives. This book, then, isn't just about happiness; it's about a way of life. Hence the title, *Full Heart Living*. This book is about living in a particular, full-hearted way that promotes a profound sense of personal contentment and happiness.

As you may have experienced, happiness can be contagious. So it was for me in conducting the interviews. Simply being in the presence of these very happy people boosted my own spirits. Furthermore, talking with happy folks about what happiness is and how to cultivate it lifted both their spirits and mine even more. Interviewing the happiest people I know for this book, in fact, is a prime example of practicing the number one component of Full Heart Living: enhancing relationships. The people I interviewed know how important it is to create and keep connections. They make family and friends a top priority. They take time to be with people they love—and they get loads of love in return. Furthermore, I learned from them that making the most of relationships with others enhances my relationship with myself; I can't help but get more in touch with my own thoughts and feelings as I'm preparing for and in the midst of meaningful encounters. So my heart extends both to others and myself—and grows in the process. Another great lesson I learned is that the more meaningful our encounters and the deeper our connections, the happier we become.

Because we intentionally came together to talk about something vitally important to us—how to be happy—conducting the interviews for this book created some very real connections. Seeing how powerful connecting with others can be, I'm more deliberate about creating and maintaining relationships with others in my life. I work at staying in touch with folks with whom I share a connection and care about. I plan gatherings with local friends and family for coffee, a meal, or a show, and I set aside time to Skype with or message those farther afield. I extend my heart to myself as well, trying to be as kind and compassionate with me as I would to anyone else I care about.

Another essential component in Full Heart Living is having a deep engagement in beloved activities. The people I interviewed find what brings them joy, and they do lots of it. Each and every happy person I interviewed has a passion or two: I think of Jenn's photography and found-object sculptures, Tracy's fitness work with children, and Ryan's filmmaking and rock climbing. And how about Gretchen's glorious singing? I get chills when I hear her. All my interviewees are committed to helping others. When we do what we love in the service of the greater good, happiness is multiplied exponentially. I've returned to my love of performing. Preparing to perform takes creativity and teamwork that bring me great joy. As I rehearse and perform, I focus in part on how our individual and collective efforts help others, even if it's simple things such as helping someone with a tricky dance step or lifting the audience's spirits. Because my mind and body are fully engaged, my thoughts don't wander into unproductive worry or memories as much. Therefore, I'm much less apt to miss precious moments.

"Tuning in," in fact, is another key in Full Heart Living. My interviewees all possess exceptional awareness of themselves and their surroundings. Philip and Barry might call it "waking up," while Warren says "presence," and Mia prefers "mindfulness." Whatever they call it, happy people are here right now and not somewhere else in their minds. They resist mindlessness. They notice. They are fully present to themselves and to others. For me to foster that kind of presence, I've increased my formal meditation time to about 45 minutes every day. I do so first thing, before anything else, to prime my mind. From there I try to drink in every moment of the day, being as fully present to all of it as I can. This includes the drudgery of certain household chores, the pain of a twisted ankle or the boredom of waiting in line at the store, as well as the perfect sunset and the candlelight dinner.

My interviewees don't disregard the hard parts of life. In fact, they deeply feel even so-called "negative emotions" such as sadness; this openness helps them learn from life's inevitable challenges and setbacks. They forgive, move on, and keep going. They do not minimize their feelings, nor do they brood over them or ruminate. Like most people, a part of me wants to avoid the less-than-pleasant. When I fell on a tree root while running the other day, after a few choice expletives and brushing off the dirt, I took a breath and allowed myself to experience the pain in my swelling palms and scraped-up knees. Miles from home, not a soul in sight, I acknowledged the sharp, bitter tang of momentary loneliness that was far more responsible for my tears than the physical hurt. Ironically, opening fully to these moments helps them pass more quickly—and to appreciate how well my body recovers when the pain starts to subside.

It was clear from listening to each interviewee's story that every single one had experienced as much pain and as many disappointments as anyone else. But because they choose to wholly experience all their emotions, they let themselves fully feel the emotional impact of any setbacks. Embracing even difficult feelings leaves them open and able to pay more attention to the good stuff. I know first hand what they mean. When Candy, an adorable Wheaten Terrier and my constant 16-year companion, died, I let myself feel the grief, trusting that in time I'd feel better. While it took months, eventually, I did feel better. In the meantime, some friends didn't appreciate that I was less fun to be around. Despite that, and hard as it was to endure, I allowed myself to stand in and then move through the natural process of mourning. All the good Candy brought me is more than worth it. Welcoming and being with the grief allowed me to fully let her go. Then I was able to appreciate again the good in the here and now. I doubt that happens when we do the stiff upper lip thing.

Likewise, my interviewees experience the fullness of the happy times, too! They wholeheartedly embrace joy. When we open to all of life, including the dull and painful, not only can we more easily see what is right for us, we can also more completely appreciate the good. Less happy people tend to dampen pleasant experiences as well as unpleasant ones. Chances are that when they were young, important adults in their lives may have said it's not good to brag, or that flying high will only lead to making it worse when things inevitably turn sour. My interviewees know that's a bunch of hooey. Why not get all you can out of the good times while they are right here?

All my interviewees are grateful. In various ways, they express their thanks frequently, whether to a higher power or to those they encounter, silently or aloud. I am not as consistent as I'd like in that, but I try to remember to breathe a silent word of thanks before eating or drinking. Throughout the day, I take random moments to think how grateful I am for my spouse, our amazing son, and our loving families and friends. I am grateful for our health and home and neighbors, the beauty of the light in autumn, the life all around in our garden. If we tried, I bet we'd find that the list of things to be grateful for is infinite.

Another important factor in living happy is creating a strong, healthy personal foundation by practicing self-care. My interviewees tend to eat less junk food and move their bodies more than the average bear. They engage in activities that calm them. They don't abuse alcohol and other drugs. They obtain adequate relaxation and sleep. They seek medical help if and when they need it. I've been pretty good in this area for years— throughout most of my adult life, in fact. I visit trusted healthcare professionals regularly and follow their advice (most of the time, at least). In addition to getting decent rest and sleep, meditating daily and exercising nearly every day, under the advice of an integrative doctor, I take supplements to balance my mood and reduce anxiety.

Good self-care includes self-acceptance, a trait I find in spades in my interviewees. They are less conforming and may even appear quirky, such as Jenn always dressing in a tie and man's cap or Barry wearing shorts at professional meetings. Because they accept themselves, they're able to take more risks and attribute any so-called "failures" to circumstances instead of some inherent bad in their very constitution. Taking more risks increases their odds of finding things that bring happiness. Self-acceptance frees up energy to pursue passions (worrying about how bad we are and trying to be perfect wastes a lot of energy). My interviewees accept and are true to themselves, warts and all. For me, acknowledging and accepting that, like Mia, I am highly sensitive and tend toward the anxious is an example of self-acceptance.

In doing this project, I learned that I might never be able to arrive at a definition of happiness that will satisfy others. I can say, however, that the happier people I interviewed tend to do a number of similar things. Of all the wonderful insights, tips, and tools, these for me have meant the most:

1. Happier people connect with themselves. They know who they are, they're true to themselves, and they're aware of their thoughts and feelings. They don't find that they are too distracted to appreciate the present moment.
2. They connect with others. They are involved in communities in which they care about others and feel cared about in return.
3. They engage in activities they are passionate about, and when those activities improve the lives of others, they are even happier.

Since I had the tremendous opportunity to glean these insights, I have worked hard to incorporate them into my own life. Every day, I attempt to connect with myself, spend time with loved ones, and do things I love, particularly in the service of a higher good. I am far from perfect, and I'm getting better at believing I am okay even when I make mistakes. I am still learning.

I've also come to appreciate the paradoxical nature of happiness. Happiness does not mean never being down or never having a bad day. Rather, happier people embrace the wholeness of life—the good and the bad, the happy and the sad. By knowing when I'm sad, and not avoiding it or squelching it, I'm far more able to appreciate the times when I'm not sad. I no longer expect to be happy every day.

My interviewees also helped me see that happiness is a process, not a destination. Much like a car needs oil changes and other regular upkeep, happiness needs ongoing attention to sustain it. Such maintenance starts with a clear intention. My interviewees all made a conscious decision to be happy, each in their own way. Then they took on their own maintenance plan. Use the following worksheet now to begin to plan your next steps toward Full Heart Living. Start wherever you like.

You know happy people, too. They're everywhere! You just have to look, to notice, to ask. So look, notice, and ask! Nearly everyone I asked was willing, eager, and honored to talk about happiness, even in front of a video camera. Meet some of them for yourself at http://www. fullheartliving.com. Reflecting on what makes them happy seemed to affirm and solidify their happiness.

Why not do the same by finding your own interview subjects? Identify who in your life appears happy. Keep it simple. You don't have to videotape them or write a book about what you learn if you don't want to! Just listen. Ask questions, and genuinely hear what they say—with a full heart. And then, please, join the larger conversation. Share with others what you learn from your conversations with the happiest people you know. You can also tell me about it here [https://www.facebook.com/fullheartliving/]. I'd love to hear from you.

MY FULL HEART LIVING PLAN:

ACTION	A FEW POSSIBILITIES
Decide	Declare your intention
	Write it in a journal
	Tell a trusted friend
	Place reminders in prominent places
Connect	Journal thoughts and feelings
	Make a date with a friend
	Give the cashier eye contact
	Forgive someone
Cultivate mindfulness	Learn to meditate
	Take yoga, Tai Chi, or qigong classes
	Fully attend to whatever is happening right now
Engage your passions	Start (or return to) a hobby
	Make a "bucket list"
	Serve others
Take care of yourself	
Eat better	Stop eating and drinking junk
	Eat whole foods, but not too much
	Add an additional vegetable each day
Move your body	Go for a 10-minute walk
Get rest	Schedule & take downtime
Express gratitude	Say thank you, both silently and aloud
	Keep a gratitude journal
Accept yourself	Determine what can and can't be changed
	Hold yourself with kindness
Develop resilience	(do all of the above and below!)
Consume news in moderation	Take news fasts
Take risks	Feel the fear, and do it anyway
Persist	Break projects into manageable pieces
	Avoid taking setbacks personally
	Find alternative ways to reach your goal
Live with intention	Choose to be happy
Embrace meaning	Volunteer
	Attend a spiritual service
Play	Do something just for fun
Laugh	See a comedy
Talk about happiness	Hang with the happiest people you know
	Ask them what they do
	Share what you learn with others

WHAT I DO NOW

MY NEXT STEPS

EPILOGUE

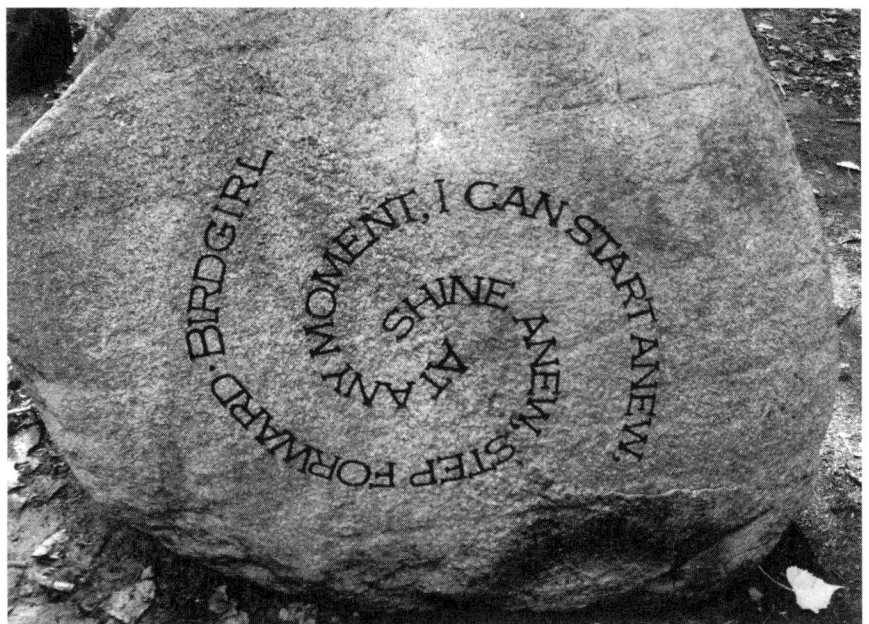

Thirteen boulders in the woods

The Twin Cities are famous for miles of biking and walking trails that surround and connect our many lakes. Of all these many trails, my favorites are the lesser-known, unpaved "hidden" hiking paths on the east side of Cedar Lake, which abound with wildlife and mature trees. Though in reality the city center is less than two miles away, here I feel I'm in another world.

This wilderness is especially beautiful in the summer when its green canopy envelops, welcomes, and protects, causing me to imagine I'm in nature's cathedral. A spiritual teacher once told me that being in nature is a form of meditation, as nature doesn't judge. I couldn't agree more. Here, I breathe deeply and feel at peace. Places like this seem to invite magic.

Over the past few years, I have noticed all sorts of remarkable art in these woods—huge sculptures made from fallen branches and logs or large stones stacked precariously one atop another. These anonymous artists' offerings give new meaning to found art, especially since these structures eventually give way to the elements. I feel awed and inspired when I encounter these beautiful expressions of creativity.

A few years ago, I discovered a more permanent artist installation while out running one sunny, early spring day. It was the first time I had been around the lake since the previous fall. I wasn't in the best of moods that morning; I'd just received word that I was not cast in a musical I'd had my heart set on. But my disappointment was dwarfed by thoughts of self-doubt. While I was cutting through the neighborhood that leads to the trails, my old self-talk started in with, "I'm too old to be returning to this acting thing," and "Maybe I'm not as talented as I thought." And, for added measure, "I sure don't have thick enough skin for all this rejection." To combat these harsh words, I tried bringing myself to the present moment by focusing on my running and the beauty all around me, but their effect lingered.

I entered the unpaved portion of the trail proper and soon was deep into the woods. Here, the lake on my left was barely visible through the thick trees that were just beginning to sprout new buds. I continued running, still trying to shake off my discontent, when suddenly, as the trail turned left, I stopped cold in my tracks. There to the side of the trail, where I was sure the previous fall only a few lonely, fallen branches, rotting logs and scattered leaves had lain, was an astounding sculpture. Thirteen boulders were carefully arranged in the shape of a spiral. At the spiral's end, the smallest rock measured about a foot in diameter. Each successive boulder increased in size, culminating with the center stone that was some three feet in diameter. I stared in wonder at this extraordinary arrangement. Had it always been here? Could I have missed it on my previous runs?

After a few moments, I was drawn to the equally astounding words chiseled into the center stone, also arranged in a spiral. They read: "At any moment, I can start anew, shine anew, step forward." ~Bird Girl

It was one of those moments when everything in the universe seems to click into place. I felt completely empowered to do whatever I wanted to do. Bird Girl's message instantly transformed my mood. It's not too late! The opportunity is here, now! Whether I'm cast in any particular musical doesn't matter in the long run. Whatever happens, with or without acting, I have a rich, full, happy life. All I have to do is follow my heart and keep on taking the next step forward.

After I returned home, I started asking around to see if anyone knew about Bird Girl and her rock sculpture. Eventually, I was told "Bird Girl" was the nickname of a wise old crone who had lived near these woods for many years. Before she moved away the previous winter, she left a lasting testament to the woods she clearly loved as much as I do. That's all I was able to discover. What was her real name? Where did she go? Is this her only sculpture? The rest remains a mystery, but Bird Girl clearly aimed to inspire generations to come.

I often have reflected on the simple yet profound words Bird Girl left behind. At any moment, we can start again. And not just start over; I hear her urging us to let our light shine and to step forward in it.

Bird Girl knows we're ready. She believes it, and so do I. So join me in the dance of happiness. No matter where you are, no matter how you feel now, at any moment, you, too, can start anew. Go ahead. Breathe in and out deeply. Take that first, full-hearted step.

Resources and
Suggestions for Further Exploration

Books

Anderson, Susan *The Journey from Abandonment to Healing*

Aron, Elaine *The Highly Sensitive Person*

Brach, Tara *Radical Acceptance: Embracing Your Life With the Heart of a Buddha*

Bridges, William *Transitions*

Brown, Brené *Daring Greatly: How the Courage to Be Vulnerable Transforms the Way We Live Love, Parent, and Lead*

Brown, Brené *Rising Strong: The Reckoning, The Rumble, The Revolution*

Cain, Susan *Quiet: The Power of Introverts in a World that Can't Stop Talking*

Cameron, Julia *The Artist's Way*

Chodron, Pema *When Things Fall Apart*

Chodron, Pema *The Wisdom of No Escape*

Chrowley, Chris and Harry Lodge, M.D. *Younger Next Year*

Csikszentmihalyi, Mihaly *Flow: The Psychology of Optimal Experience*

Diamandis, Peter H. and Steven Kotler *Abundance*

Dominguez, Joe and Vicki Robin *Your Money Or Your Life*

Elias, Maurice J., et. al. *Emotionally Intelligent Parenting*

Emmons, Henry *The Chemistry of Calm*

Emmons, Henry *The Chemistry of Joy*

Emmons, Henry, et. al. *The Chemistry of Joy Workbook*

Emmons, Robert *Thanks! How the New Science of Gratitude can make you Happier*

Feldman, David B. & Lee Daniel Kravetz *Supersurvivors*

Frederick, Ron *Living Like You Mean it: Use the Wisdom and Power of Your Emotions to Get the Life you Really Want*

Fromm, Eric *The Art of Loving*

Goleman, Daniel *Emotional Intelligence*

Gottman, John *The Relationship Cure*

Gottman, John *The Seven Principles for Making Marriage Work*

Hanh, Thich Nhat *How to Love*

Harris, Dan *10% Happier: How I Tamed the Voice in My Head, Reduced Stress Without Losing My Edge, and Found Self-Help That Actually Works—A True Story*

Hlava, Patty *Cultivating Gratitude*

Hlava, Patty *Living Gratitude*
Kabat-Zinn, Jon *Coming to Our Senses*
Kabat-Zinn, Jon *Full Catastrophe Living*
Kabat-Zinn, Jon *Wherever You Go, There You Are*
Kornfield, Jack *The Art of Forgiveness, Lovingkindness, and Peace*
Lyubormirsky, Sonja *The How of Happiness*
Myers, David *The American Paradox: Spiritual Hunger in an Age of Plenty*
Ricard, Matthieu *Happiness: A Guide to Developing Life's Most Important Skill*
Rubin, Gretchen *The Happiness Project*
Rumi, Jalal Al-Din, Coleman Barks (translator) *The Illuminated Rumi*
Seligman, Martin E.P. *Authentic Happiness: Using the New Positive Psychology to Realize Your Potential for Lasting Fulfillment*
Seligman, Martin E.P. *Learned Optimism: How to Change Your Mind and Your Life*
Servan-Schreiber, David *Anti-Cancer: A New Way of Life*
Siegel, Ronald D. *The Mindful Solution: Everyday Practices for Everyday Problems*
Snyder, C.R. and Shane J. Lopez *Positive Psychology: The Scientific and Practical Explorations of Human Strengths*
Vanzant, Iyanla *Peace from Broken Pieces: How to get through What You're going through*
Weisberg, Andy *Laid Off and Crazy Happy*
Ywahoo, Dhyani *108 Quotations*
Ywahoo, Dhyani *Learning Cherokee Ways*
Ywahoo, Dhyani *Voices of Our Ancestors*

Online

My Blog www.facebook.com/fullheartliving/
Happiness Webisodes: www.fullheartliving.com
Videos, research, self tests and more: http://www.authentichappiness.sas.upenn.edu/Default.aspx
Happiness Tracker: https://www.trackyourhappiness.org/
Marelisa Fabrega 22 Gratitude Exercises That Will Change Your Life http://daringtolivefully.com/gratitude-exercises
Heart-to-Heart Couples Retreats http://heart.mn.cx

Research

Comparative effectiveness of exercise and drug interventions on mortality outcomes: metaepidemiological study
BMJ 2013; 347 doi: http://dx.doi.org/10.1136/bmj.f5577 (Published 01 October 2013) *British Medical Journal* 2013;347:f5577

The anti-inflammatory effect of exercise
Anne Marie W. Petersen , Bente Klarlund Pedersen
Journal of Applied Physiology Published 1 April 2005 Vol. 98 no. 4, 1154-1162

Physical Activity and the Prevention of Depression: A Systematic Review of Prospective Studies, George Mammen, MSc, Guy Faulkner, PhD, *American Journal of Preventive Medicine,* Volume 45, Issue 5, November 2013, Pages 649–657

J Leukoc Biol. 2005 Oct;78(4):819-35. Epub 2005 Jul 20.

Physical activity and modulation of systemic low-level inflammation.

Bruunsgaard H1.

Bruunsgaard H. Physical activity and modulation of systemic low-level inflammation. *Journal of leukocyte biology* 2005; 78: 819-35.

Calder PC, Kew S. The immune system: a target for functional foods? *The British journal of nutrition* 2002; 88 Suppl 2: S165-77.

Appendix

Tests

I didn't choose my interviewees only because they said they were happy or seemed happy to me. I wanted some sort of objective criteria to back up my choices and dispel critics. Not wanting to ask too much of my subjects, I asked them to answer a few brief surveys.

First I asked folks to rate themselves on a 10-point happiness scale, where 10 is the happiest they can imagine. Their answer had to be 9 or 10. Next, I asked them to complete Giltay's Optimism Questions, Diener's Satisfaction With Life Scale, and The Flourishing Scale (FS) by Diener and Biswas-Diener. Interviewees also completed Martin Seligman's online 24-item Authentic Happiness Inventory Questionnaire and reported their score to me. (The only exception to taking these tests was my expert, Dr. Emmons.)

Authentic Happiness Inventory Questionnaire

It's free. http://www.authentichappiness.sas.upenn.edu/Default.aspx

For further information on Giltay's Optimism Questions, please see:

Giltay EJ, Kamphuis MH, Kalmijn S, Zitman FG, Kromhout D. Dispositional optimism and the risk of cardiovascular death: the Zutphen Elderly Study. *Archives of Internal Medicine* 2006;166:431-6.

Rius-Ottenheim N, Kromhout D, van der Mast RC, Zitman FG, Geleijnse JM, Giltay EJ. Dispositional optimism and loneliness in older men. *International Journal of Geriatric Psychiatry*. 2012;27:151-9.

The Satisfaction with Life Scale (SWLS) is in the public domain (not copyrighted); therefore, you are free to use it without permission or charge by all professionals (researchers and practitioners) as long as you give credit to the authors of the scale: Ed Diener, Robert A. Emmons, Randy J. Larsen and Sharon Griffin as noted in the 1985 article in the *Journal of Personality Assessment*.

Diener, E., Emmons, R. A., Larsen, R. J., & Griffin, S. (1985). The Satisfaction with Life Scale. *Journal of Personality Assessment*, 49, 71-75.

Pavot, W. G., Diener, E., Colvin, C. R., & Sandvik, E. (1991). Further validation of the Satisfaction with Life Scale: Evidence for the cross-method convergence of well-being measures. *Journal of Personality Assessment*, 57, 149-161.

Pavot, W., & Diener, E. (1993). Review of the Satisfaction with Life Scale. *Psychological Assessment*, 5, 164-172.

Pavot, W., & Diener, E. (2008). The Satisfaction With Life Scale and the emerging construct of life satisfaction. *Journal of Positive Psychology*, 3, 137–152

The Flourishing Scale (FS) is copyrighted but you are free to use it without permission or charge by all professionals (researchers and practitioners) as long as you give credit to the authors of the scale:

Diener, E., Wirtz, D., Tov, W., Kim-Prieto, C., Choi, D., Oishi, S., & Biswas-Diener, R. (2009). New measures of well-being: Flourishing and positive and negative feelings. *Social Indicators Research*, 39, 247-266.

Full-Hearted Appreciation

Countless souls contributed to the realization of this book.

- Special acknowledgment goes to Barry, Gretchen, Jenn, Mia, Philip, Tracy, Ryan, Warren, and Dr. Henry Emmons.
- Jamie Anderson, Nancy Anderson, Rachel Anderson, Sarah Bergstrom, Candace Barrett Birk, Mary Bonner, Stephen Cohen, Bill Cooper, Jr., Eva Chava Curland, Cheri Desmond-May, Kathi Dunn, Nadine Emerson, Jac Enge, Laurie Beth Fitz, Linda Gallaher, Ana Hagedorn, Patty Hlava, Hobie Hobart, R.D. Hutchins, Thérèse Jacobs-Stewart, Cindy Kaiser, Kyoko Katayama, Paige Mann, Joe Mann, Bob Marcus, Dorie McClelland, Sharon Stein McNamara, Mary Carroll Moore, Kit Naylor, Mame Pelletier, Mykel Ann Pennington, Roxanne Sadovsky, Heidi Schneider, Vicky Swedenburg, Doug Toft, Carol Valenti, Elizabeth Wexler, Nicole Marie Wilder, and Merra Young deserve special thanks.
- Marilyn Ruby's contributions warrant extra special thanks. Wow.
- Miss Collier (aka Jan Manino), my fifth grade Baldwin Elementary teacher. You told me I am an author and I believed you.
- My editor, Barb Chintz: you made me laugh while cajoling and never coddling. What wonders you have done.
- A thousand thanks to all my family and friends. I couldn't be without you.
- I would also like to acknowledge the gratitude I feel for my clients who open themselves so courageously and from whom I learn so much.
- Most of all, thank you Muse, invisible guides from beyond, the wellspring of creativity and inspiration.

Index

Brickman, P. D., 31
Buddhism
  awareness and acceptance
    in, 204
  Radical Acceptance, 63
  10,000 joys and 10,000
    sorrows, 122
bullying, 5–7, 17–18, 91–
  93. *See also* reactions
burnout, 162–163

C
Cain, Susan, 190
calming the mind
  breathing for, 94
  increased awareness,
    201–205
  resiliency, 126–127
  stress reduction, 37
  See also meditation
Cameron, Julia, 135–136
Campbell, Donald T., 31
change, 48
characteristics of happy
  people, 33, 218, 239–242
Chodron, Pema, 118
choices
  capacity for, 155–156
  deliberate, 32
  focus on immediate
    benefits, 49
  food, 45–46, 138
  monitoring thoughts
    and, 79
  news media exposure,
    139
  priority of happiness,
    182
  purposeful, 201–202
  seeing the good in
    others, 205
conflict in relationships
  between couples,
    107–110
  soft start-up in, 114
  taking responsibility for,
    112
  work, 106
  See also relationships
connecting with others,
  101–114. *See also*

relationships
conscious living. *See*
  mindfulness
consciousness. *See*
  mindfulness
contentedness, 20
Crowley, Chris, 39–42
Csikszentmihalyi, Mihaly,
  87
cytokines, 39–41

D
Darran, 199–200
decelerate. *See* calming the
  mind
deliberate choices. *See*
  choices
depression, 47–48, 51, 87,
  121, 123, 132n. *See also*
  bipolar disorder
determination, **199–209**
  active decision for
    change, 200
  Darran's milestone, 199
  decelerate for awareness,
    202–205
  decide, 199–201
  remind, 201
  See also choices
developing mindfulness.
  See mindfulness
Diamandis, Peter H., 136
disposition. *See* Highly
  Sensitive People
distractions, 54, 81, 96,
  111, 138, 162
doubts, 162–163

E
embracing difference,
  189–198
  aquarium visit, 189
  self-talk, 193
  self-validation, 194
  sensitivity, 189
Emmons, Henry
  awareness for choices,
    201
  be who I am, 15–16
  brain changes in
    awareness, 33

choice toward happiness,
  203
cultivating mindfulness,
  80
distractions, 139
epigenetics, 33
fatty acids and, 46–48
formal practice for, 80
joy, 121–123
karma, 202–203
nutrition and movement,
  45–46
risk taking, 169
sadness/grief, 77–78
Seven Roots of
  Resilience, 124–130
Emmons, Robert, 64
emotional intelligence
  (EQ), 9, 113
emotional paralysis, 157
emotions
  awareness and
    unpleasant, 202
  chronic emotional stress,
    39–40
  connection to thoughts,
    78
  with gratitude, 66
  inner coding of, 203–
    204
endorphins, 37, 39
energy
  anger, 155
  anxiety, 184
  management, 124
environment, 31–32
epigenetics, 33
euphoria, 38–39, 51
exercise. *See* physical
  activity
expressing thanks, **59–74**

F
failure
  associated feelings, 173
  finding passion, 213
  learning opportunity
    from, 171–172
  risk taking and fear, 169
  See also shame; success
false "I don't know," 157

mood, 43, 45–46, 125, 139
resilience and, 123, 132n
smart food tips, 52–54
whole foods, 42–43

O
obligation, 149
obliviousness, 75. *See also* mindfulness
obsession, 155
omega fatty acids, 46–47
open-heartedness, 128
opportunity, 21–23. *See also* risk taking
optimism, 11
overcoming shame. *See* shame
Owen, 228
oxytocin, 67

P
pain
endorphins and perception of, 37
happiness from, 237
healing with validation of, 117
passion, 85–90
creating connections, 213–214
discovery of, 85–87
signs of happiness, 10
passive-aggressive behavior, 5
passiveness, 155, 157
patience, 62–63
Patty, 65–66, 68
peace and tranquility, 21
perfectionism, 78–79
perseverance, 155–156
Personal Reflection/ Couple Dialogue (PR/ CD), 108–110
perspective
alcohol effects, 43
interpretation of the world, 23–24
maintaining, 26, 130
passion in, 85–90
scarcity mindset, 66

Philip
attention with travel, 79
awareness of surroundings, 76
career aligned with values, 182, 186
ebb and flow of life, 23
internal sensations, 182
mindfulness, 76, 79–80
nutrition, 43
obsessive about happiness, 12–13
physical activity
boosting immunity, 124
concentration with, 38, 82–83
foundation for happiness, 43
gene activation, 82–83
immediate benefits, 50
managing energy, 124–125
mood and, 38, 47–48
promoting good sleep, 126
running, 41–42
self-care, 36, 132
Positive Psychology, 8
projection, 105
protecting yourself, 135– 142. *See also* news media

Q
quotations
Antoine de Saint-Exupéry, 238
Bird Girl, 250
EM Foster, 128–129
Fran Kafka, 77
George Orwell, 195
George Sand, 101
Rumi, 88, 91
Thich Nhat Hanh, x

R
Radical Acceptance, 62, 70
reactions
awareness of, 95, 205
awareness of emotional, 201
defined, 94

highly sensitive people, 192
to passive-aggressive person, 4–5
response to actions of others, 97
thoughts and sensations, ix
reading vacation, 136
realism, 23
rejection
persistence with, 172
personal, 168
physiological response, 116
self-talk with, 250
relationships
communications in, 110
contact in, 103–104
50th birthday party discussion, 105–108
self-acceptance and exposure in, 104–105
toxic, 1–7
See also conflict in relationships
relaxation
energy management, 130
guided full body, 126
self-care and calming, 132, 206
sleep, 55
resentment
blame with, 38
demonizing other with, 120
with focus on self, 69
lashing out with, 108
volunteering, 149–150, 152
resilience, 115–133
affirmations of self, 163
being in the moment/ present, 118
connecting with others, 128–129
mental roots of, 126
self-care and, 123–124
Seven Roots of Resiliency, 124–130
success and, 172